The Low-GI Slow Cooker

The Low-GI Slow Cooker

Delicious and Easy Dishes Made Healthy with the Glycemic Index

DR. MARIZA SNYDER, DR. LAUREN CLUM AND ANNA V. ZULAICA

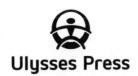

Ulysses Press

Published in the U.S. by
ULYSSES PRESS
P.O. Box 3440
Berkeley, CA 94703
www.ulyssespress.com

ISBN13: 978-1-61243-180-2
Library of Congress Control Number 2013931793

Acquisitions Editor: Kelly Reed
Managing Editor: Claire Chun
Project Editor: Alice Riegert
Editor: Susan Lang
Proofreader: Barbara Schultz
Index: Sayre Van Young
Cover design: what!design @ whatweb.com
Production layout: what!design @ whatweb.com
Cover photos: grilled fish and vegetables © Anna Hoychuk/shutterstock
    .com; brussels sprouts © Peredn15ankina/shutterstock.com; seafood
    stew © HLPhoto/shutterstock.com; pumkin custard © Edith Frinco/
    shutterstock.com

Printed in the United States by Bang Printing
10 9 8 7 6 5 4 3 2 1

Distributed by Publishers Group West

NOTE TO READERS
This book has been written and published strictly for informational and
educational purposes only. It is not intended to serve as medical advice or to be
any form of medical treatment. You should always consult your physician before
altering or changing any aspect of your medical treatment and/or undertaking
a diet regimen, including the guidelines as described in this book. Do not stop
or change any prescription medications without the guidance and advice of
your physician. Any use of the information in this book is made on the reader's
good judgment after consulting with his or her physician and is the reader's
sole responsibility. This book is not intended to diagnose or treat any medical
condition and is not a substitute for a physician.

This book is dedicated to our families,
for their ongoing love and support,
and to all of you that are consistently striving to make healthy changes!

Contents

Introduction

Dear Sugar,

I'm breaking up with you. You're no good for me. You make me sluggish and moody, I don't sleep as well and you affect my workouts. So while we've had some fun, and you are delicious, I have to cut you off. Perhaps we'll run into each other from time to time, but you CANNOT come over every night anymore.

Good-bye, Sugar.

This cutesy "Dear John" breakup letter to sugar was a Facebook post by Dr. Lauren Clum several years ago. It was intended to be an amusing way to get people to think about their own sugar consumption, yet it actually began a significant process of self-discovery for the author. It brought awareness to the concept of sugar addiction that pervades our culture and society, and piqued an interest in helping people to understand how sugars and carbohydrates affect their bodies and health. The glycemic index (GI) is the perfect tool to assist in this understanding, as it rates foods based on how quickly they're absorbed by the body after consumption, and how a given food affects blood sugar. Using this tool as a guide for meal planning is an easy way to ensure healthy eating.

If you're perusing this book, you're probably well aware that two of the biggest public health issues facing our society today are insulin resistance and diabetes. Currently, diabetes is the fastest growing chronic disease. It is estimated that approximately 80 million children and adults in the United States have diabetes or are on the verge of developing the disease. This statistic is alarming and even scary, but it doesn't have to continue! Type 2 (adult-onset) diabetes and insulin resistance are avoidable and even reversible with proper dietary practices and exercise.

Eating low-GI foods such as fruits and vegetables, along with healthy fats and proteins, can help reverse chronic disease, especially type 2 diabetes. Diets that include low-GI foods have been shown to regulate both lipid and glucose levels in people diagnosed with type 1 (insulin-dependent) and type 2 diabetes. Recent studies from the Harvard School of Public Health have shown that a low-GI food-based diet offers significant benefits for weight control, diabetes, and coronary heart disease.

SECTION 1

Getting Started

Chapter 1

What Is the Glycemic Index?

We live in a time where there is no shortage of information about weight loss and healthy eating, yet much of that information is conflicting and confusing. Various and extreme diets—from those that cut carbohydrates to ones that cut fat, and everything in between—reign supreme, whether or not they're healthy or effective. In general, people are not exactly sure what healthy carbohydrates and fats are, or if they even exist, and they may be surprised to learn that eating foods containing them can actually help keep weight off and bodies healthy. It's time to dispel myths once and for all and approach healthy eating in a different way.

We are not advocating a diet but rather a lifestyle filled with nutrient-dense foods that nourish the body and soul. Many people have followed a fad diet in the past, sometimes several times over, and many have experienced temporary weight loss. Often the weight comes back on just as quickly as it came off, and people find themselves in a vicious cycle of yo-yo dieting, with steady weight gain as the result. We know how frustrating it can be trying to figure out how to lose excess fat and sustain long-term weight loss once and for all. Utilizing the glycemic index as a tool to understand how the human body processes carbohydrates can help people make decisions to help them achieve their health and weight-loss goals.

Scientists who research how the body digests carbohydrates tell us that not all carbohydrates are created equal and that we must not completely avoid carbohydrates, particularly the ones in vegetables and fruits. Carbohydrates are vital for body and brain functions, as they contribute to glucose, the required fuel for the proper functioning of the brain, muscles, red blood cells, and organs. Significantly decreasing carbohydrate intake can be dangerous to health because when glucose reserves become too low, the body is forced to break down amino acids for fuel instead of using them for more vital functions.

Exactly how carbohydrates affect the digestive system and blood sugar levels can now be measured. This information is meant to empower people to make more intelligent choices about what they put into their bodies. As a tool, the glycemic index can educate people on which carbohydrates to consume in generous portions and which to consume less frequently.

Keep in mind that the most important carbohydrates—the ones that should never be avoided—are vegetables and fruits rather than grains. Fruits and vegetables are healing foods that contain antioxidants, vitamins, and minerals necessary for biological function, and that help to prevent chronic diseases. Vegetables and fruits are the carbohydrates that should be consumed in large quantities on a daily basis, and they are the basis of the recipes in this book.

The GI Research Service (SUGiRS), established at Australia's University of Sydney in 1995, began measuring the glycemic index of foods by using strict standardized and validated scientific methods. It defines the glycemic index (GI) as the ranking of carbohydrates on a scale of 0 to 100, in accordance with which a food raises blood sugar levels 2 to 3 hours after eating. Foods with a high GI designation are those that are rapidly digested and absorbed into the body, producing high fluctuations in blood sugar and insulin levels. Low-GI foods are slowly digested and absorbed through the digestive track, producing a gradual and steady rise in insulin and blood sugar levels. These foods have been shown to have positive benefits for overall health and weight. Avoiding spikes and keeping blood sugar relatively steady help control appetite and delay hunger cues, additionally aiding in weight management.

Many people are under the impression that plain table sugar and desserts are the culprits that people with insulin resistance and/or diabetes must avoid, but glycemic index research proves otherwise. Complex carbohydrates, like starchy potatoes and rice, cause a high spike in blood sugar. A general understanding of the types of carbohydrates that spike blood sugar and raise insulin levels allows people to limit such foods. Utilizing the glycemic index as a reference tool can ensure healthier food choices and lead to healthy weight loss.

The University of Sydney's GI Research Service's glycemic index (www.glycemicindex.com) does not promote a specific weight-loss diet plan or label carbohydrates as good or bad. Rather, it recommends that the glycemic index be used as a tool to help choose which foods to eat, and it provides the following suggestions:

- Focus on breakfast cereals based on barley, oats, or millet.
- Choose breads made with whole grains, stoneground flour, or sourdough.
- Eat fewer servings of potatoes and rice.
- Eat an abundance of fruits and vegetables.
- Avoid processed carbohydrates, such as pasta.

The GI value of a food cannot be guessed by simply looking at the composition of the food. It must be calculated at designated laboratories to determine how the body's blood sugar level responds.

Foods tested for categorization within the glycemic index are given scores:

- High: >70. Examples include white and brown rice, bread, and red and white potatoes.
- Medium: 56–69. Examples include corn, bananas, pineapple, raisins, and dates.
- Low: <55. Examples include carrots, apples, grapefruit, peas, nonfat milk, kidney beans, lentils, and peanuts.

Because carbohydrates tend to be consumed in combination with other foods at a meal, the glycemic load (GL) was created to give a more complete picture of how carbohydrate consumption affects blood sugar levels after a full meal. Glycemic load is a ranking system for food that measures the amount of carbohydrates in a serving of food. Calculating the glycemic load of a meal is the most practical way to apply information from the glycemic index to everyday healthy eating. Glycemic load is calculated by multiplying a particular food or recipe's glycemic index by the number of net carbohydrates in a given serving and dividing by 100. Net carbohydrates are equal to the total grams of carbohydrates in a serving, minus the grams of dietary fiber for that serving.

$$GL = (GI \times Net\ Carbs) \div 100$$

The glycemic load provides a good indication of how much that serving of food is likely to increase your blood sugar levels. Foods or servings with GL values below 10 are considered to have a low impact on blood sugar levels; foods with a GL value between 11 and 19 have a moderate impact; and GL values above 20 are considered high and cause blood sugar levels to spike. Just because a meal has medium- or even high-GI foods in it doesn't necessarily mean that the GL will be high. Both the glycemic index and glycemic load are listed for each and every recipe in this book. Flipping through the recipes will reveal how a particular combination of ingredients may affect the glycemic load. You'll see how small amounts of medium- or high-GI ingredients can still create a low-GL meal. Because the GL is related to the meal's effect on blood sugar levels, low-GL meals are often recommended for controlling insulin resistance, diabetes, and weight.

While the glycemic index is a tool rather than a diet, the simple fact is that everyone can benefit by eating whole foods that contain a balance of proteins and healthy fats, and that are lower on the glycemic index. Foods with a lower GI and GL are typically higher in fiber and other nutrients, providing you with nourishment and making you feel full. These foods are broken down more slowly in the digestive system, allowing for proper nutrient absorption and a steadier influence on blood sugar. The result is that you feel full longer and have more energy.

We have always advocated eating real food, keeping whole food nutrition simple, and utilizing tools such as the glycemic index to better understand what's going into our bodies. Cross-referencing foods that are low on the glycemic index with those that are known for their superfood capabilities yields a list of the same foods! For instance, known superfoods such as kale, blueberries, beans, and oats have low GI and GL values. The foods that have well-known healing capabilities are the ones that are more slowly broken down by the body, the ones that steadily affect blood sugar instead of spiking it.

In each of our books we have emphasized the importance of eating real food. In this era of convenience, grocery stores are lined with processed foods and filled with non-food ingredients that contribute to the growing incidence of chronic diseases in our families and communities. There are more than 20,000 cheap, foodlike products pretending to be real food in the standard grocery store. These foodlike substances are far from real food, with the bulk of their ingredients being highly processed wheat, corn, soy, sugar and/or unpronounceable additives. Most all of these highly processed foods have very high GI and GL values, indicating that they cause significant spikes in blood sugar when consumed. Many of the ingredients found specifically in processed carbohydrate-based products spike blood glucose and insulin levels. Over time, these dramatic fluctuations lead to insulin resistance and the potential development of chronic conditions such as type 2 diabetes and heart disease.

The recipes in this book call for good-quality, whole food ingredients that are easy to find and filled with vital nutrients to yield healthy meals, including desserts. When choosing ingredients, look for fresh, local, organic produce, dairy, meat, grains, and herbs. The soil in which food is grown impacts the final product; organic produce is grown in vitamin- and mineral-rich soil. If you can't find organic produce, buy fresh and local produce, and rinse it thoroughly to remove impurities before use.

Be wary of any packaged goods. Just because a packaged food product says it has a low GI score does not necessarily mean it is healthy. It does not mean that it isn't, either, so ask yourself: Can I pronounce and recognize all of these ingredients? Are there five or fewer ingredients listed? Get in the habit of reading ingredient lists and labels, and remember that the best foods to put into your body typically contain only one ingredient and do not even have labels, namely fruits and vegetables. Each individual fruit or vegetable boasts its own unique combination of health benefits, so be sure to eat a variety—aim for all the colors of the rainbow to get the full spectrum of essential nutrients.

If we could only give 10 tips for improving health, aside from using the glycemic index as a tool, this is what we'd suggest.

1. To get the greatest amounts of key nutrients from your fruits and veggies, buy what's in season.

2. Stock your kitchen with healthy convenience foods, cut up veggies, hummus, raw nuts, and fruit, to avoid bingeing on unhealthy, high-GI snacks.

3. Double up your serving of veggies. One cup of veggies equals two servings.

4. Have fresh berries and other fruits for dessert to satisfy your sweet tooth.

5. For a quick snack or breakfast, choose organic plain yogurt with raw sliced almonds and fresh fruit.

6. Stock up on heart-healthy raw nuts to give your entree or salad a boost of crunch and healthy fat.

7. Drink plenty of water throughout the day. Keep water with you at all times—at work, in the car, at the gym—and always drink it during meals.

8. Eat the colors of the rainbow at every meal.

9. Get a boost of protein and healthy fat by making your coffee or latte with almond milk.

10. Green smoothies made with almond milk, fresh fruit, and greens are a fast way to maximize servings of fruits and veggies in any meal.

Chapter 2

Myths and Science Behind Nutrition

In helping people learn to make healthy choices, one of our biggest duties is to bust the myths about health and nutrition, and there are quite a few out there! There are many misconceptions about what is or isn't healthy when it comes to food and eating, and it is our goal with this book not only to shed light on this confusing topic, but to simplify the whole process of choosing healthful foods.

Myth #1: The glycemic index is a diet. The first thing to remember is that the glycemic index is a tool, not a diet. The index is simply a categorization of foods, particularly carbohydrates, to show how a given food affects blood sugar. By understanding which foods spike blood sugar more than others, you can make healthier choices about which ingredients to use in recipes. However, just because a food is higher on the GI doesn't mean that it has to be avoided completely! The most important rule for healthy eating is to eat real food. So if a food is high on the GI but is not processed and is a real food, then it can still be utilized, just not in every recipe that you make. Use lower GI foods liberally, and higher GI foods more sparingly.

Myth #2: The glycemic index is a treatment.   No, the glycemic index is not a treatment. Healthy eating is something that everyone can and should employ, regardless of whether or not they're facing a health challenge. Unfortunately, often people are more inspired to make healthy changes when they face a health problem, or when they've been diagnosed with a specific condition such as diabetes, hypertension, irritable bowel syndrome, ulcerative colitis, or cancer. And it is at this point that healthy eating is of the utmost importance to encourage healing. But the GI is an effective tool for healthy eating at any point, not just when there's cleanup to do! So it shouldn't be seen as a treatment to use when health has hit rock bottom, but as a tool to utilize to make healthy choices in order to promote health before it becomes compromised.

Myth #3: Health problems are hereditary.   This is a very important myth to bust, as all too often genes are unnecessarily blamed for unhealthy habits. People will quickly point to a family history of degenerative conditions to explain away why they, too, have a particular condition. However, most degenerative conditions arise in response to habits and behaviors, not solely because of genetics. Often the reason that a certain degenerative condition is perceived to be hereditary is because generation after generation will employ similar habits and behaviors that lead them down similar health paths. For example, the foods that we eat and how we prepare them are often learned in childhood, and carried on from generation to generation. If we were raised eating a certain food or preparing a meal a certain way, that is how we will continue eating into adulthood, and we're likely to pass the same habits and behaviors on to our children. The same goes for exercise: If you were raised with exercise as an everyday part of life, you're more likely to continue the habit of exercising into adulthood. Similarly, people who don't exercise will suffer the health consequences, just as generations before them who didn't exercise faced similar consequences. Understanding these concepts can empower people to make different, perhaps healthier choices than in the past or than other family members. These choices can then influence their health picture, despite family history of disease. The GI can help guide these choices.

Myth #4: All fats are bad.   This myth is one of the unhealthiest of them all! Fat is absolutely necessary for health, and cannot be omitted from a healthy diet. Fat has gained a terrible reputation in the past 30 years of the low-fat medical craze in our society and as a result is horribly misunderstood. The reality is, every cell in the body is lined with fat, and healthy fat is essential to maintain the function of those cells. Cutting fat out of the diet is a surefire way to decrease cell function, which leads to all sorts of health issues.

However, all fats are not created equal, which is why the subject causes so much confusion. The healthiest fats come from real food sources, whether they're unsaturated or saturated fats. Yes, even saturated fats can be healthy! The most important thing is to look at the source of the fat—if it comes from a real food, it can be healthy. Fats are not listed on the GI, as they do not have carbohydrates or sugar in them. It is up to each person to look at where a fat is coming from, and whether or not it should be included in a meal plan. Healthy fats can be found throughout the recipes in this book, so use them as a guide to which fats to use. When healthy fats are paired with low-GI foods, amazingly delicious and healthy meals emerge. As a rule, trans fats should always be avoided.

Myth #5: All carbohydrates are the same.   Over the past 30 years, as our society became more and more fearful of fats, carbohydrates gained popularity because of their low fat content. However, the increase in carbohydrates was not healthy, either. All carbohydrates break down to sugar in the body, so regardless of how little fat a carbohydrate has, it still acts like sugar physiologically. As people cut the fat and increased the sugar (carbohydrates) in their diets, their cells and bodies suffered the consequences, resulting in an astonishing increase in degenerative health conditions. The GI has proven to be an excellent tool in helping people make smart decisions regarding carbohydrates. Because fruits and vegetables are carbohydrates, it's not okay to just cut carbs from our diets. But it is necessary to understand them, which is where the glycemic index comes in. The GI depicts how much a given food and its carbohydrates affect blood sugar, so that people can make smarter decisions about what they choose to put in their bodies.

Myth #6: Health is just about numbers.   Simply put, health is greater than the sum of its parts. It's not enough to simply look at the breakdown of different foods, from carbohydrates and fats to various nutrients, to understand whether a certain food is a healthy choice. Numbers can be manipulated, and simply because a food is labeled with low or high numbers in certain categories doesn't necessarily make it healthy to eat. This is why the most basic food rule that we teach is: eat real food. Preparing your meals with ingredients that are real food is the absolute best way to know what exactly is going into your body.

In dispelling some common myths, we broadly discussed carbohydrates and fats. Now let's break them down into a little more detail. Carbohydrates, also known as starches and sugars, are commonly understood to be utilized by the body for fuel.

They break down to form glucose, which the body uses as energy to maintain healthy brain, muscle, blood cell and organ function. Carbohydrates that don't get turned into glucose for fuel get stored as fat, so it is very important that their intake be controlled. The most important carbohydrates to consume are in the form of fruits and vegetables, with their incredibly valuable vitamin and mineral content. However, fruits and vegetables still break down as sugar in the body, and each fruit and vegetable is not created equal. The glycemic index categorizes fruits and vegetables by how they affect blood sugar after consumption, and the ones that break down more slowly and get absorbed through the digestive tract should dominate your diet.

The desirable vitamins and minerals within fruits and vegetables cannot be absorbed by the body without adequate fat consumption. Healthy fats allow for improved absorption of vitamins and minerals. If your fat intake is inadequate, your body will not absorb vital nutrients, regardless of how many fruits and vegetables you consume. The recipes in this book include a variety of healthy fats not only for flavor, but also to support proper absorption of the carbohydrate-based ingredients in the recipes.

As long as they are available, carbohydrates will be utilized for fuel by the body. However, any sugars not used for fuel will be stored as fat—and fat is burned for fuel only when there are no longer carbohydrates for the body to use. So if a person consistently consumes lots of sugar, beyond those in fruits and vegetables, that sugar will be added to the stored fat and won't get burned.

Sugar consumption is an epidemic. Across the board, people are addicted to sugar. As with any addiction, it must be fed, and if it's not, the body will go through physiological withdrawal. Sugar has pervaded just about every processed food, so its addiction has pretty much gone unnoticed in our culture. Because nearly everyone is addicted to it, no one realizes that they are, until they try giving it up, that is. When people attempt to cut sugar from their diets, they undergo physical withdrawal, suffering from symptoms varying from headaches and low energy to the shakes and violent mood swings. As a result, the addiction is not broken very often. It's an addiction that begins in childhood, and continues over the course of a lifetime. However, it can be overcome! As with kicking any addiction, it takes dedicated commitment, a plan, and time. A plan can be created by utilizing tools like the glycemic index to better understand what is in food and which foods to put into our bodies.

In an effort to not consume too much sugar, often people will turn to artificial sweeteners. However, this is not a healthy solution at all. Aside from artificial sweeteners being just that, artificial, they are heavily processed chemicals that wreak havoc on the body. Many are neurotoxins that attack brain cells and significantly alter brain chemistry. The buildup of these toxins has been shown to increase the likelihood of many degenerative brain conditions. As such, artificial sweeteners should be avoided at all costs. The idea is to break the sugar addiction completely, not to replace the sugar with a more harmful substance.

Chapter 3

Benefits of Slow Cookers

The slow cooker is a beloved appliance in many households including ours, which is why dedicating a recipe book to it appealed to us. We went a step further and emphasized low-GI recipes to enhance the numerous benefits of the slow cooker. The many advantages of this easy cooking method extend from saving money to increasing the nutritional value of meals.

Convenience is such a valuable commodity in today's world, especially when it comes to cooking. As a society, we spend less time preparing and eating meals than our parents and grandparents did, and in the process we have sacrificed nutrition. The slow cooker brings back the benefits of a home-cooked meal without the hassle of having to constantly babysit the stovetop and oven. A slow cooker typically can be left unattended for several hours, and heat is indirectly applied to food so that it cooks evenly without any stirring or other intervention necessary. Some of the recipes in this book utilize the stovetop or oven, but the majority of cooking time uses the slow cooker. The recipes were tested in real-life conditions—amid work responsibilities, running errands, exercising, and visiting with friends and family. Using the slow cooker consistently allows people to fit everything in—working, studying, going to the gym—without missing the opportunity to prepare and eat nutritious home-cooked food.

The slow cooker is a fast favorite for home cooking, thanks to its ability to help prepare flavorful and delicious healthy foods without a lot of mess or fuss. The recipes in this book were created to maximize flavor while minimizing prep time and impact on the waistline. A slow cooker offers extreme affordability for home cooking, from energy usage to recipe ingredients. It uses the same amount of electricity as a 75-watt light bulb, considerably less energy compared with an electric oven or stovetop. Most come with a timer that enables the cooker to automatically turn the heat way down or even shut off completely once cooking has completed, using only the necessary energy for cooking. A slow cooker also transforms inexpensive ingredients such as root vegetables, grains, and tough cuts of meat into tender, flavorful dishes.

One of the greatest attributes of the slow cooker is its ability to preserve the nutritional value of the ingredients in a recipe. With traditional cooking at high temperatures, vital nutrients such as vitamins and minerals are typically degraded or even lost. Often these nutrients get cooked out of foods or thrown out with water used in cooking, decreasing the nutritional value of the meal, even when you start with ingredients that are high in vitamins and minerals. Meals prepared in a slow cooker are heated at relatively low heat for a longer period of time than food that is fried, steamed, or boiled. As with all cooking methods, there will be a breakdown of some nutrients, especially enzymes. However, slow cooking preserves more vitamins and minerals because of the lower temperatures, and nutrients are more easily recaptured in the resulting sauces or juices served with the meal. Additionally, the extended cooking time of slow-cooked meals allows for better distribution of flavors while preserving nutrients.

Home cooking allows for control over the quality of ingredients and the nutrient profile of a meal, resulting in healthier meals. Most of our slow cooker recipes are built around fresh vegetables and healthy cuts of meat, omitting processed foods that not only increase calories but are filled with toxic chemicals. When fresh, wholesome ingredients are used in slow cooking, flavor abounds without sacrificing the waistline.

With slow cooking, it's best to utilize ingredients that generally take longer to cook. Tough or dense cuts of meat, such as brisket, beef shank, or pork shoulder, are great choices. Since these cuts of meat are generally less expensive than their more tender counterparts, consider looking for organic, grass-fed options to ensure the best quality ingredients. These tougher cuts of meat, cooked slowly for many hours, become deliciously tender and fall off the bone easily. Cooking bone-in meats provides the added benefit of pulling nutrients from the bone. Hearty vegetables and low-GI grains are also great options for slow cooking. Look for crunchy root vegetables and grains that naturally take a long time to cook.

Limit the use of canned fruits and vegetables when using the slow cooker. Canned foods have already been cooked and have lost almost all their nutritional value, and in a slow cooker they often turn into tasteless mush. Just a few of our recipes call for anything other than fresh ingredients. Unless a recipe specifically calls for a canned ingredient, use fresh ingredients.

Also use fresh herbs and seasonings whenever possible. Since slow cooking involves a long, slow simmer, flavor can often be lost throughout the cooking process. That's why we use lots of fresh herbs and spices to heighten the flavors of the dishes. Sometimes we'll recommend toasting or roasting herbs and spices before adding them to the slow cooker—please pay attention to these details to ensure the success of each meal!

Aside from minimizing prep time, a slow cooker aids convenience by using just one pot! Washing pots and pans is often last on the list of desirable things to do after dinner, and a slow cooker goes a long way toward simplifying cleanup. It makes large family meals and holiday gatherings less daunting, and frees up the stovetop and oven for other uses.

SECTION 2

Recipes

Notes from the Chef

Here are some helpful tips on particular ingredients used throughout the recipes.

Coconut Milk: Two types of coconut milk are used in these recipes. The first is canned coconut milk, the creamier, thicker milk usually sold in a can and typically found in the international aisle of your supermarket. The second is the thinner drink version sold in boxes or cartons. Please note that coconut water is not included in any recipes and should not be used as a substitute for coconut milk.

Almond Milk: If almond milk is not readily available or too expensive for your budget, it is very simple to make at home. Soak 1 cup raw almonds in cold water for 12 to 24 hours. Alternatively, you can boil water and soak the nuts in the hot water for 30 minutes to 1 hour. Add the soaked almonds to a blender with 2 cups water and vanilla extract if you'd like. The more water you add, the runnier the almond milk will be. Adjust the thickness to your liking. Strain in a cheesecloth and enjoy!

Choosing Canned Foods: Some recipes will call for canned tomatoes, beans, or artichokes. It is very convenient to use these products, especially when we are pressed for time and wouldn't normally have time to boil, peel, and prepare an artichoke just for its artichoke hearts. When you do buy canned goods, please read the label, making sure that it is a low-sodium product. It is also recommended that you rinse beans or artichokes once you do take them out of the can, just to wash away the excess sodium and flavor that have developed from the juices it is stored in. For canned tomato sauce, it is advisable to go with the best quality your store has to offer. The flavor and texture of the tomatoes are definitely noticeable and your dish will have a wonderful flavor.

Coconut Palm Sugar: It is very difficult to create a variety of slow cooker recipes for desserts without using any sugar. After doing extensive research, we learned of a sweetener that is one of the best options for anybody on a low-GI regime. Coconut palm sugar is low on the glycemic index and high in nutrients and amino acids. If you read the ingredient list, you'll see that it's made from granulated coconut and flower blossom nectar, and no unpronounceable chemicals or ingredients. Your local health food store should carry coconut palm sugar or you can order it online. If you are having a hard time finding coconut palm sugar, then maple sugar is an acceptable alternative, although it is a bit higher on the glycemic index.

Toasted Spices: Many of the recipes call for toasting and then grinding spices. You can toast them on a baking sheet in the oven or in a pan on the stovetop—both methods work well. The reason there are two steps is that toasting the spice will bring out the natural oils and make it very fragrant. Crushing it in a blender or processor will ensure that those oils get released in the food you are adding them to.

Toasted Nuts: Many recipes call for toasting nuts or seeds. Toasting the nuts or seeds helps release the natural oils inside, and the flavor becomes a bit more profound. There are a couple of methods to toast nuts or seeds. Heat a large dry skillet over high heat, and add the nuts or seeds when the pan is hot. Shake the pan often until the nuts or seeds start to brown and become fragrant, about 2 to 3 minutes. Remove and set aside to prevent from burning. Another method of toasting them is to toast them in the oven. Preheat your oven to 400°F. Spread the nuts or seeds on a baking sheet and place in the oven for 3 to 4 minutes, stirring the nuts or seeds once. Once they have browned and are fragrant, remove from the oven and remove from the baking sheet to prevent them from burning.

Browning and Searing Meat: Many recipes call for searing meat prior to placing it in the slow cooker. By searing meat, you are caramelizing the outside of the meat, which in turn will release more flavor into the other ingredients in the slow cooker. Searing is not essential to the success of a recipe, but it is recommended. Browning ground meat in a hot pan also helps to caramelize the meat and add more flavor to the slow cooker ingredients. It also allows for the fat to be released from the meat so you can easily drain it off before adding the meat to the slow cooker. Browning ground meat also makes the meat look more appetizing after it is fully cooked.

Chapter 4

Breakfast

When most people think of slow cooker recipes, they don't think of breakfast dishes. But, yes, you can indeed make delicious breakfast dishes that are low GI! In this section, we use whole grains and steel cut oats, since it takes the body longer to break them down and they produce a steady stream of sugar in the body rather than a spike. Eggs are delicious made in the slow cooker—just make sure to check them by inserting your knife, as a slow cooker sometimes has a mind of its own. Also, grease the inside of the slow cooker with nonstick cooking spray, olive oil spray, or your favorite oil anytime you are cooking eggs.

Polenta Breakfast Casserole

Serves 4

¼ cup chopped white onion

1 cup yellow cornmeal

3 cups water

4 large eggs

2 tablespoons grated Parmesan cheese

¼ teaspoon cracked black pepper

2 cups packed arugula

1 teaspoon extra virgin olive oil

1 tablespoon red wine vinegar

1 teaspoon salt

Spray the inside of the slow cooker with nonstick spray.
Add the onion, cornmeal, and water to your slow cooker.
Cover and cook on high for 1 hour. Remove the lid and
stir to even out the polenta. Carefully crack one egg at a
time onto the outer part of the polenta, until you make a
circle with the four eggs. Top with the Parmesan cheese
and cracked black pepper, and put the lid back on. Cook
on high for an additional 20 minutes. Turn the heat off, but
leave the lid on. Check the consistency of the yolks after 5
minutes and serve when they are to your liking.

Meanwhile, in a medium bowl, toss together the arugula,
olive oil, and vinegar, and season with the salt and more
pepper taste. For each serving, scoop out polenta with one
egg and top with ½ cup tossed arugula.

Serving size: ½ cup cooked polenta, 1 egg, ½ cup tossed arugula	
Each serving	
Glycemic Index	Medium
Glycemic Load	14
Calories	219
Fat	9 g
Saturated Fat	3 g
Carbohydrates	25 g
Fiber	3 g
Protein	11 g

Creamy Peach and Almond Quinoa

Serves 4

½ cup pre-rinsed quinoa*

1½ cups water

1½ cups plain, unsweetened almond milk

¼ cup toasted sliced almonds

⅓ cup fresh or frozen peaches, cut into ¼-inch pieces

2 tablespoons golden raisins

¼ teaspoon almond extract

⅛ teaspoon sea salt

Combine all the ingredients in your slow cooker, and stir well. Cover and cook on low for 4 to 6 hours or on high for 2 to 2½ hours, or until the quinoa has fully sprouted. Uncover and let the quinoa sit for 10 minutes to set before serving.

* Read the label on your quinoa to see if it is pre-rinsed. Even if it is pre-rinsed, make sure to rinse it again through a fine-mesh strainer until the water runs clear. Quinoa is naturally coated in saponin, a bitter, resinlike coating.

Serving size: ½ *cup*	
Each serving	
Glycemic Index	Medium
Glycemic Load	9
Calories	148
Fat	5 g
Saturated Fat	0.2 g
Carbohydrates	22 g
Fiber	3 g
Protein	5 g

Spicy Oatmeal
Serves 4

1 cup steel cut oats

4½ cups water

¼ teaspoon ground cinnamon

⅛ teaspoon ground ginger

⅛ teaspoon ground nutmeg

2 tablespoons raisins

4 tablespoons toasted walnut pieces

Combine all the ingredients in your slow cooker, and stir well. Cover and cook on low for 5 to 6 hours or on high for 2½ to 3 hours, or until the oats have absorbed all the liquid and are creamy. The raisins in this dish give the oatmeal a touch of sweetness and the walnuts provide a bit of texture.

Serving size: ½ cup cooked oatmeal, 1 tablespoon walnuts	
Each serving	
Glycemic Index	Medium
Glycemic Load	14
Calories	197
Fat	8 g
Saturated Fat	1 g
Carbohydrates	30 g
Fiber	5 g
Protein	7 g

French Toast Casserole
Serves 4

FRENCH TOAST

4 slices sprouted grain bread, such as Ezekiel 4:9 flax bread

3 large eggs

½ cup coconut milk

½ cup plain, unsweetened almond milk

¼ cup unsweetened applesauce

½ teaspoon ground cinnamon

⅛ teaspoon ground nutmeg

½ teaspoon vanilla extract

TOPPING

4 tablespoons pure maple syrup

2 tablespoons hot water

⅛ teaspoon ground cinnamon

¼ cup chopped walnuts

Spray the bottom of your slow cooker with a nonstick spray. Cut each bread slice in half diagonally and shingle the triangles in two rows or one row (depending on the size of your slow cooker) in the slow cooker. In a large bowl, whisk the eggs, coconut milk, almond milk, applesauce, cinnamon, nutmeg, and vanilla extract. Pour over the top of the shingled bread slices, making sure to wet them evenly.

In a small bowl, mix together the ingredients for the topping and drizzle over the bread mixture. Cover and cook on low for 3 to 4 hours or on high for 1 to 1½ hours, until the wet mixture has set.

Serving Suggestion: Enjoy with fresh fruit, such as strawberries and blueberries, or with eggs on the side.

Serving size: *2 triangles French toast (1 slice sprouted grain bread), 1 teaspoon walnuts*

Each serving	
Glycemic Index	Low
Glycemic Load	13
Calories	251
Fat	10 g
Saturated Fat	2 g
Carbohydrates	30 g
Fiber	4 g
Protein	10 g

Lemon Ricotta Breakfast Soufflé with Raspberries

Serves 6

½ cup almond meal

¼ cup oat flour

⅓ cup coconut palm sugar

¼ teaspoon salt

4 large eggs, separated

⅔ cup whole ricotta, drained in cheesecloth or on paper towels
  for at least 30 minutes

2 tablespoons melted coconut oil

¼ cup lemon juice

zest of 1 lemon

¼ teaspoon vanilla extract

¼ cup raspberries

Combine the almond meal, oat flour, sugar, and salt in a medium bowl. Mix together the egg yolks, drained ricotta, melted coconut oil, lemon juice and zest, and vanilla in a large bowl, whisking until the ingredients are incorporated and the batter is smooth. Add the flour mixture to the egg yolk mixture, and whisk until smooth.

Place the egg whites in a mixing bowl and beat with an electric mixer until stiff peaks form. Add a small dollop of the whipped egg whites to the batter and mix it in to lighten the batter. Add the remaining whipped egg whites in two batches and gently fold in with a spatula until combined.

Lightly grease the bottom and lower sides of the slow cooker with nonstick spray. Pour in the batter and lightly scatter the raspberries on the top of the batter. Lay two paper towels over the top of the slow cooker, place the lid on top of the paper towels, and cook on low for 1½ to 2 hours, or until an inserted knife comes out clean.

Serving size: 3 ounces	
Each serving	
Glycemic Index	Low
Glycemic Load	4
Calories	258
Fat	18 g
Saturated Fat	8 g
Carbohydrates	20 g
Fiber	2 g
Protein	10 g

Almond Oatmeal

Serves 4

1 cup steel cut oats

4½ cups unsweetened almond milk

4 tablespoons toasted sliced almonds

Combine the oats and almond milk in your slow cooker.
Cover and cook on low for 5 to 6 hours, or until the oats
have absorbed all the liquid and are creamy. Sprinkle each
serving with 1 tablespoon of almonds.

Serving size: ½ cup cooked oatmeal, 1 tablespoon almonds	
Each serving	
Glycemic Index	Low
Glycemic Load	12
Calories	219
Fat	9 g
Saturated Fat	0.7 g
Carbohydrates	30 g
Fiber	6 g
Protein	8 g

Very Berry Barley

Serves 6

1 cup hulled barley*

3½ cups water

¾ cup blackberries

¾ cup quartered strawberries

Combine the barley, water, blackberries, and strawberries in your slow cooker. Cover and cook on low for 3 to 4 hours or on high for 1 to 2 hours or until the barley is soft but still has texture to it. Cooked barley should not be mushy; it should have a bit to it.

Serving Suggestion: Enjoy with a drizzle of maple syrup or toasted walnut pieces.

* Check the label on the barley. If it is "unhulled barley," then you will have to soak it overnight in water and then cook it.

Serving size: ½ cup	
Each serving	
Glycemic Index	Low
Glycemic Load	3
Calories	47
Fat	0.3 g
Saturated Fat	0 g
Carbohydrates	11 g
Fiber	2 g
Protein	0.8 g

Savory Zucchini and Sweet Potato Torte with Chive Sour Cream
Serves 4

ZUCCHINI AND SWEET POTATO TORTE

1 pound zucchini, grated (about 2 cups packed)

1 small unpeeled sweet potato, grated (about ¾ cup packed)

¼ cup grated onion

1 large clove garlic, minced

4 large eggs, beaten

¼ teaspoon sea salt

⅛ teaspoon red pepper flakes

¼ teaspoon cracked black pepper

CHIVE SOUR CREAM

¾ cup low-fat sour cream

1 tablespoon finely chopped chives

½ teaspoon lemon juice

Lightly spray the inside of your slow cooker with nonstick spray. Place the grated zucchini in the center of a kitchen or tea towel. Fold one side up and roll into a log. Tightly twist both ends to wring out any liquid. Place the drained zucchini in a large bowl, add the sweet potato, onion, garlic, eggs, salt, red pepper flakes, and black pepper, and mix well. Pour the mixture into the slow cooker, and spread it out evenly, using a spatula or your hands. Cover and cook on low for 2½ to 3 hours or on high for 50 minutes to 1 hour, or until the eggs have set and an inserted knife comes out clean.

To make the chive sour cream, whisk together the sour cream, chives, and lemon juice. Store in the refrigerator until the torte is cooked. Drizzle 1 tablespoon over the top of each serving.

Serving size: *4 ounces torte, 1 tablespoon sauce*	
Each serving	
Glycemic Index	Low
Glycemic Load	16
Calories	206
Fat	14 g
Saturated Fat	7 g
Carbohydrates	13 g
Fiber	3 g
Protein	9 g

Sausage Frittata

Serves 4

1 cup precooked Italian sausage (about 2 links), chopped into
  ¼-inch pieces

4 large eggs

4 egg whites

¼ cup 1% milk

¼ teaspoon dried basil

⅛ teaspoon red pepper flakes

½ teaspoon sea salt

¼ teaspoon cracked black pepper

Spray the inside of your slow cooker with nonstick spray.
Add the chopped sausage and spread it into an even layer.
In a medium bowl, combine all the remaining ingredients
and whisk well. Pour the egg mixture over the sausage,
making sure to distribute it evenly. Cover and cook on low
for 2½ to 3 hours or on high for 45 minutes to 1 hour, or
until the eggs have set. Cut into wedges with a spatula and
scoop out.

Serving size: *1 4-ounce wedge*	
Each serving	
Glycemic Index	Low
Glycemic Load	1
Calories	199
Fat	14 g
Saturated Fat	5 g
Carbohydrates	2 g
Fiber	0 g
Protein	18 g

Vegetable Frittata with Pecorino Shavings

Serves 6

1 cup thinly sliced zucchini

½ cup chopped red bell pepper

1 cup roughly chopped broccoli florets

2 large cloves garlic, minced

8 large eggs, beaten

½ cup grated mozzarella cheese

¼ cup shaved pecorino Romano cheese

1 teaspoon sea salt

½ teaspoon cracked black pepper

½ cup minced fresh flat-leaf parsley

Spray the inside of your slow cooker with nonstick spray. Lay the zucchini slices to completely cover the base of the slow cooker. Sprinkle the bell pepper, broccoli, and garlic over the zucchini. In a large bowl, whisk the eggs, cheeses, salt, and black pepper. Pour the egg and cheese mixture over the vegetables, but do not stir it in. Cover and cook on low for 3 to 3½ hours or on high for 1½ to 2 hours, or until the eggs have set and an inserted knife comes out clean. Sprinkle each serving with chopped parsley.

Serving size: *1 4-ounce wedge*	
Each serving	
Glycemic Index	Low
Glycemic Load	1
Calories	178
Fat	11 g
Saturated Fat	5 g
Carbohydrates	4.6 g
Fiber	1.3 g
Protein	16 g

Chapter 5

Soups

Among the easiest dishes to prepare in the slow cooker, soups can be made in large batches for a party, to last throughout the week, or to freeze for future use. In this chapter you will find vegetarian, vegan, and meaty soups to suit your cravings and needs, and all consist of whole foods packed with nutrients and flavor. These soup recipes are perfect for starting in the slow cooker right before you run errands or leave for work.

Chicken Broth

Makes 4 quarts (12 cups)

1 small chicken carcass or bones from a 3- to 4-pound bird,
  skin and meat removed

½ large white onion, roughly chopped

3 large carrots, roughly chopped

3 celery stalks, roughly chopped

2 bay leaves

1 bunch fresh thyme

1 bunch fresh oregano

1 tablespoon black peppercorns

8 large cloves garlic

4 quarts (12 cups) water

Preheat the oven to 500°F or the broiler to high. Lay out
the bones on a rimmed baking sheet that has been lined
with parchment paper. Bake or broil for 4 to 5 minutes, or
until the bones start to brown. Place the onion, carrots, and
celery in your slow cooker, and put the baked or broiled
chicken bones on top, breaking the carcass if it's too tall.
Add the bay leaves, thyme, oregano, peppercorns, and
garlic. Pour in the water, adding more if necessary to cover
the chicken bones. Cover and cook on low for 10 to 12
hours (preferable) or on high for 4 to 5 hours. Strain and
cool the liquid, discarding the bones, vegetables, and herbs.
Cool overnight, and the next day use a fine sieve to remove
any fat that has settled at the top.

Chef's Tip: Do not add any salt to the broth. This will allow
for more control of your sodium intake and of the flavor of
the foods you add the broth to.

Serving size: *1 cup*	
Each serving	
Glycemic Index	Low
Glycemic Load	0
Calories	15
Fat	0 g
Saturated Fat	0 g
Carbohydrates	1 g
Fiber	0 g
Protein	2 g

Vegetable Broth
Makes 4 quarts (12 cups)

½ large white onion, roughly chopped

3 large carrots, roughly chopped

1 small leek, green part and root end removed, white part
washed well and roughly chopped

3 celery stalks, roughly chopped

2 bay leaves

1 bunch fresh thyme

1 bunch fresh oregano

1 tablespoon black peppercorns

8 large cloves garlic

4 quarts (12 cups) water

Preheat the oven to 500°F or the broiler to high. Lay out
the onion, carrots, leek, and celery on a baking sheet lined
with parchment paper. Bake or broil for 4 to 5 minutes, or
until the vegetables start to brown. Remove from the oven
and place in your slow cooker. Add the bay leaves, thyme,
oregano, peppercorns, and garlic. Pour in the water. Cover
and cook on low for 10 to 12 hours (preferable) or on high
for 4 to 5 hours. Strain and cool the liquid, discarding the
vegetables and herbs. Cool overnight, and the next day use
a fine sieve to remove any fat that has settled at the top.

Chef's Tip: Do not add any salt to the broth. This will allow
for more control of your sodium intake and of the flavor of
the foods you add the broth to.

Serving size: *1 cup*	
Each serving	
Glycemic Index	Low
Glycemic Load	0
Calories	15
Fat	0 g
Saturated Fat	0 g
Carbohydrates	1 g
Fiber	0 g
Protein	2 g

Beef Broth

Makes 4 quarts (12 cups)

1 pound beef bones with lots of marrow, such as knuckle and
tail bones

½ pound veal bones

½ large white onion, roughly chopped

3 large carrots, roughly chopped

3 celery stalks, roughly chopped

2 bay leaves

1 bunch fresh thyme

1 bunch fresh oregano

8 large cloves garlic

4 quarts (12 cups) water

Preheat the oven to 500°F or your broiler to high. Line a
rimmed baking sheet with parchment paper and lay out the
bones. Bake or broil for 4 to 5 minutes, or until the bones
start to brown. Place the onion, carrot, and celery in your
slow cooker, and put the roasted bones along with any
juices that may have been released on top of the vegetables.
Add the bay leaves, thyme, oregano, and garlic. Pour in the
water. Cover and cook on low for 10 to 12 hours. Strain and
cool the liquid, discarding the bones, vegetables, and herbs.
Cool overnight, and the next day use a fine sieve to remove
any fat that settled at the top.

Chef's Tip: Do not add any salt to the broth. This will allow
for more control of your sodium intake and of the flavor of
the foods you add the broth to.

Serving size: *1 cup*	
Each serving	
Glycemic Index	Low
Glycemic Load	0
Calories	20
Fat	0 g
Saturated Fat	0 g
Carbohydrates	1 g
Fiber	0 g
Protein	3 g

Spicy Iranian Chicken Stew

Serves 4

1 tablespoon extra virgin olive oil

2 tablespoons chopped white onion

4 large cloves garlic, thinly sliced

12 ounces boneless, skinless chicken breasts, trimmed of fat,
  cut into bite-size pieces

¼ teaspoon sea salt

¼ teaspoon ground black pepper

1 (8-ounce) can tomato sauce

¼ cup low-sodium chicken broth (recipe on page 54)

1 (15-ounce) can garbanzo beans, drained and rinsed

1 large jalapeño pepper, cut into thin rounds, deseeded if less
  heat is desired

¾ cup loosely packed, de-stemmed, roughly chopped dill

1 cup loosely packed, de-stemmed, roughly chopped cilantro

1 teaspoon curry powder

½ teaspoon turmeric

¼ teaspoon ground cumin

In a medium sauté pan over medium heat, heat the oil.
Add the onion and garlic, and cook until the onion is
translucent, about 2 to 3 minutes, then place in the slow
cooker. In a small bowl, season the chicken with the salt
and pepper, and toss to coat. Transfer to the slow cooker,
and add the tomato sauce, chicken broth, garbanzo beans,
jalapeño, dill, cilantro, curry, turmeric, and cumin, and mix
well. Cover and cook on low for 3 to 4 hours or on high for
1½ to 2 hours, or until chicken easily pulls apart.

Serving size: *3 ounces chicken, ¼ cup garbanzo beans with sauce*	
Each serving	
Glycemic Index	Low
Glycemic Load	11
Calories	277
Fat	4 g
Saturated Fat	0.8 g
Carbohydrates	34 g
Fiber	7 g
Protein	27 g

Chicken Sausage and Kale Soup

Serves 6

½ teaspoon fennel seeds

1 small yellow onion, diced

2 large carrots, quartered and chopped

2 large cloves garlic, minced

1 cup de-stemmed, roughly chopped lacinato or dino kale, divided

12 ounces precooked chicken sausage, cut into ½-inch half moons

6 cups low-sodium chicken broth (recipe on page 54)

¼ teaspoon red pepper flakes

Sea salt, to taste

Cracked black pepper, to taste

Toast the fennel seeds: Heat a small sauté pan over medium to high heat, and add the seeds when the pan is hot. Shake the pan constantly, until the seeds are fragrant, about 2 to 3 minutes. Pulse the seeds in a food processor or blender and set aside.

Place the onion, carrots, garlic, ½ cup kale, and sausage in the slow cooker. Add the chicken broth, red pepper flakes, and fennel seeds, and cover. Cook on low for 7 to 8 hours or on high for 4 to 5 hours. Remove the lid and ladle half of the soup into a blender. Puree, then return to the slow cooker. Add the remaining ½ cup kale, cover, and with the setting on high, cook an additional 10 to 15 minutes, or until the kale is tender. Season with salt and pepper to taste.

Serving size: *1 cup*	
Each serving	
Glycemic Index	Low
Glycemic Load	1
Calories	154
Fat	9 g
Saturated Fat	2 g
Carbohydrates	11 g
Fiber	2 g
Protein	9 g

Veggie Chili
Serves 8

4 cups low-sodium chicken broth (recipe on page 54)

1 (15-ounce) can garbanzo beans, drained and rinsed

1 (15-ounce) can black beans, drained and rinsed

2 (15-ounce) cans kidney beans, drained and rinsed

1 (15-ounce) can diced tomatoes

2½ cups chopped zucchini

1 large red bell pepper, chopped

½ cup chopped red onion

2 celery stalks, finely chopped

1 tablespoon chili powder

¼ teaspoon ground cumin

½ teaspoon dried parsley

½ teaspoon dried oregano

½ teaspoon dried basil

3 large cloves garlic, minced

1 tablespoon tomato paste

2 tablespoons extra virgin olive oil

⅛ teaspoon cracked black pepper

⅛ teaspoon sea salt

Combine all the ingredients in your slow cooker, and mix well. Cover and cook on low for 8 hours or on high for 4 hours, adding water or more broth if the chili is too dry for your liking.

Serving size: *1 cup*	
Each serving	
Glycemic Index	Low
Glycemic Load	11
Calories	306
Fat	5 g
Saturated Fat	1 g
Carbohydrates	52 g
Fiber	17 g
Protein	16 g

Albondigas Soup

Serves 4, Makes 12 to 13, 1½-inch meatballs

1 pound lean ground beef

1 tablespoon uncooked white rice

1 small Roma tomato, grated (about 1½ tablespoons)

¼ large white onion, grated (about 2 tablespoons)

2 large cloves garlic, minced

1 large egg, beaten

½ teaspoon sea salt

½ teaspoon cracked black pepper

1 medium, unpeeled sweet potato, cut into ½-inch cubes
  (about 1 cup)

3 large carrots, cut into ¼-inch rounds (about 2 cups)

2 large zucchini, cut in half and then cut into ¼-inch thick
  slices (about 3 cups)

6 cups low-sodium chicken broth (recipe on page 54)

⅛ teaspoon dried oregano

1 large bay leaf

In a large bowl, combine the ground beef, rice, grated tomato, onion, garlic, and egg. Season with salt and pepper. Using your hands, mix the ingredients until fully incorporated. Grab a pinch of the meat mixture and roll it into a 1½-inch ball. Set the meatballs on a baking sheet or plate as you make them. After you've rolled the meatballs, place the sweet potato, next the carrot, and then the zucchini in the slow cooker. Gently lay the meatballs on top of the zucchini, making sure to leave at least ½ inch between them. Add the broth, oregano, and bay leaf. Cover and cook on low for 8 to 10 hours or on high for 4 to 6 hours, or until the meatballs are no longer pink in the center and the rice is cooked through.

Serving size: *1 cup soup, 3 meatballs*	
Each serving	
Glycemic Index	Low
Glycemic Load	8
Calories	437
Fat	25 g
Saturated Fat	10 g
Carbohydrates	25 g
Fiber	5 g
Protein	27 g

Mushroom Barley Soup
Serves 6

2 tablespoons extra virgin olive oil

¼ cup chopped white onion

3 cloves garlic, minced

2 cups thinly sliced crimini mushrooms

2 cups thinly sliced portobello mushrooms, stems removed and
  gills scooped out

1 cup hulled barley

6 cups low-sodium vegetable broth (recipe on page 56)

½ teaspoon dried thyme or 1 teaspoon chopped fresh thyme

⅛ teaspoon red pepper flakes

1 teaspoon sea salt

In a large sauté pan over medium heat, heat the oil. Add the onion, garlic, and mushrooms, and cook for 5 to 6 minutes, or until golden brown. Add to the slow cooker along with the remaining ingredients, and cook on low for 7 to 8 hours or on high for 3 to 4 hours.

Serving size: *1 cup*	
Each serving	
Glycemic Index	Low
Glycemic Load	2
Calories	121
Fat	5 g
Saturated Fat	1 g
Carbohydrates	16 g
Fiber	3 g
Protein	3 g

Vegetable Miso Soup
Serves 8

8 cups water

½ cup light miso paste

8 ounces baby bok choy, quartered and chopped into
  1-inch pieces

8 ounces shiitake mushrooms, very thinly sliced

¼ cup wakame seaweed or shredded nori

¼ cup thinly sliced green onion, divided

dash of soy sauce or tamari (optional)

Combine the water and miso paste in the slow cooker and
whisk well to incorporate the miso paste. Add bok choy,
mushrooms, seaweed or nori, and half of the green onion
to the slow cooker. Cover and cook on low for 5 to 6 hours
or on high for 2 to 3 hours. Garnish each serving with the
remaining green onion and a dash of soy sauce or tamari
if using.

Serving size: *1 cup*	
Each serving	
Glycemic Index	Low
Glycemic Load	0
Calories	20
Fat	0.3 g
Saturated Fat	0.2 g
Carbohydrates	3 g
Fiber	0.5 g
Protein	2 g

"Cream" of Mushroom Soup

Serves 6

2 cups thinly sliced button mushrooms

2 cups thinly sliced crimini mushrooms

2 tablespoons extra virgin olive oil

1 large shallot, finely chopped

3 tablespoons chopped fresh flat-leaf parsley, plus 2
   tablespoons for garnish

1 tablespoon chopped fresh thyme

2 large cloves garlic, minced

½ teaspoon sea salt

½ teaspoon cracked black pepper, additional to taste

1 cup cashew butter

1 tablespoon nutritional yeast

5 cups low-sodium vegetable broth (recipe on page 56),
   divided

½ cup water

Preheat the oven to 400°F. In a large bowl, toss the button
and crimini mushrooms with the olive oil, shallots, 3
tablespoons parsley, thyme, garlic, salt, and pepper. Line
a baking sheet with parchment paper and spread out the
seasoned mushrooms in a thin layer (making sure they're
not crowded will help them brown rather than steam and
release liquid). Roast for 4 to 5 minutes, or until golden
brown. Remove from the oven and set aside.

Add the cashew butter, nutritional yeast, and 1 cup broth to
your slow cooker and whisk to mix well. Add the remaining
4 cups broth, water, and the roasted mushrooms and
shallots, then cover and cook on low for 4 to 5 hours or on
high for 2 to 3 hours, checking the soup periodically and
whisking it if there are any lumps of the cashew mixture

that have not broken up. Once the soup is cooked, use an immersion blender or upright blender to puree half the soup, and stir together the pureed and unpureed portions. Garnish each serving with cracked black pepper and a pinch of the reserved chopped parsley.

Serving size: 1 cup	
Each serving	
Glycemic Index	Low
Glycemic Load	2
Calories	232
Fat	14 g
Saturated Fat	2 g
Carbohydrates	20 g
Fiber	4 g
Protein	9 g

Broccoli and Pumpkin Seed Bisque

Serves 4

¾ cup pumpkin seeds, divided

1 tablespoon extra virgin olive oil

½ cup chopped yellow onion

2 large cloves garlic, minced

⅛ teaspoon red pepper flakes

1 pound broccoli, cut into small florets, stems thinly sliced

2 cups packed, fresh spinach

3 cups low-sodium vegetable broth (recipe on page 56)

1 teaspoon dry mustard

1 tablespoon Worcestershire sauce

1 tablespoon chopped fresh flat-leaf parsley

½ cup plain, unsweetened almond milk

¾ teaspoon sea salt

½ teaspoon cracked black pepper

Toast the pumpkin seeds: Heat a small sauté pan over medium heat, and add the seeds. Shake the pan often, until the seeds are golden brown and fragrant, about 2 to 3 minutes. Remove from the pan and set aside.

Heat the oil in the same pan on medium heat, and add the onion, garlic, and red pepper flakes. Cook, stirring often, until the onion is translucent, then transfer to your slow cooker. Add the broccoli, spinach, broth, dry mustard, Worcestershire sauce, parsley, and ½ cup toasted pumpkin seeds to the slow cooker, and mix well. Cover and cook on low for 8 to 9 hours or on high for 4 to 5 hours, or until the broccoli stems are very tender.

Use an immersion blender or upright blender to blend the soup until it is smooth. Whisk in the almond milk, salt,

and pepper. Ladle into serving bowls and garnish with 1
tablespoon toasted pumpkin seeds per serving.

Serving size: *1 cup, 1 tablespoon toasted pumpkin seeds*	
Each serving	
Glycemic Index	Low
Glycemic Load	1
Calories	167
Fat	7 g
Saturated Fat	1 g
Carbohydrates	21 g
Fiber	5 g
Protein	8 g

Smoky Turkey Chili

Serves 8

2 tablespoons extra virgin olive oil

8 ounces lean ground turkey

½ cup chopped red onion

3 large cloves garlic, minced

1 (15-ounce) can diced tomatoes

1 (15-ounce) can garbanzo beans, drained and rinsed

1 (15-ounce) can black beans, drained and rinsed

1 (15-ounce) can kidney beans, drained and rinsed

2½ cups chopped zucchini

3 cups low-sodium chicken broth (recipe on page 54)

1 tablespoon chili powder

¼ teaspoon ground cumin

1 teaspoon smoked paprika

1 canned chipotle pepper in adobo sauce, minced, plus 1
tablespoon adobo sauce

½ teaspoon dried oregano

⅛ teaspoon cracked black pepper

⅛ teaspoon sea salt

½ cup loosely packed chopped cilantro

In a large sauté pan over medium to high heat, heat the oil.
Add the ground turkey, onion, and garlic. Cook, stirring
constantly and breaking up large pieces of turkey with your
spatula, for 5 to 6 minutes, or until browned. Drain off any
fat or juices.

Combine the remaining ingredients except the cilantro in
your slow cooker, and add the cooked turkey, onion, and
garlic mixture. Mix well and cover. Cook on low for 7 or 8
hours or on high for 4 to 5 hours, adding more broth if the
chili becomes too dry. Serve with cilantro sprinkled on top.

Serving size: *1 cup*	
Each serving	
Glycemic Index	Low
Glycemic Load	11
Calories	282
Fat	7 g
Saturated Fat	1 g
Carbohydrates	40 g
Fiber	12 g
Protein	17 g

Grandma's Green Lentil Soup

Serves 8

4 slices bacon, cut into thin strips

2 cups green lentils

2½ quarts (10 cups) low-sodium vegetable or chicken broth
(recipes on page 56 and page 54)

2 large cloves garlic

½ cup chopped white onion

1 teaspoon sea salt

Heat a small sauté pan over medium to high heat. Add the
bacon strips and cook until golden brown, about 7 to 10
minutes. Remove from the pan and drain on paper towels.
Add the cooked bacon to the slow cooker, followed by
the remaining ingredients. Cover and cook on low for
8 to 10 hours or on high for 5 to 6 hours, or until the
lentils are tender.

Serving size: *¾ cup*	
Each serving	
Glycemic Index	Low
Glycemic Load	4
Calories	214
Fat	3 g
Saturated Fat	2 g
Carbohydrates	33 g
Fiber	13 g
Protein	16 g

Mexican Beef Stew
Serves 6

2 pounds beef shank

6 small oxtails (about 1 pound)

2 large carrots, cut into ¼-inch rounds (about 2 cups)

1 large zucchini, cut into ¼-inch rounds (about 2½ cups)

1 chayote squash, peeled, white core removed, and cut into
   1-inch pieces (about 1½ cups)

¼ medium cabbage, chopped into 1-inch strips (about 2 cups)

4 bay leaves

½ bunch cilantro

2 quarts (8 cups) low-sodium beef broth (recipe on page 58)

4 large cloves garlic

1 teaspoon sea salt

1 teaspoons cracked black pepper

Combine all the ingredients in the slow cooker. Cover
and cook on low for 9 to 10 hours or on high for 4½ to 6
hours, or until the meat is tender and easily pulls apart with
two forks.

Serving Suggestion: Serve with a lime wedge on the side and
your favorite salsa stirred in.

Serving size: *1 cup*	
Each serving	
Glycemic Index	Low
Glycemic Load	3
Calories	250
Fat	7 g
Saturated Fat	2 g
Carbohydrates	12 g
Fiber	4 g
Protein	35 g

White Bean Chicken Chili

Serves 8

1 teaspoon cumin seeds

2 tablespoons vegetable oil

½ cup chopped white onion

2 large Anaheim chile peppers, seeded and chopped

2 large cloves garlic, minced

4 (15-ounce) cans cannellini beans, drained and rinsed

8 ounces boneless, skinless chicken breasts, fat trimmed and
   cut into 1-inch cubes

1½ cups low-sodium chicken broth (recipe on page 54)

1 teaspoon minced jalapeño pepper

¼ cup loosely packed chopped cilantro

2 tablespoons green onion, green part thinly sliced

1 teaspoon sea salt

½ teaspoon cracked black pepper

Toast the cumin seeds: Heat a small sauté pan over medium
to high heat, and add the seeds once the pan is hot. Shake
the pan constantly, until the seeds are fragrant, about 1
minute. Grind the toasted seeds by pulsing them in a food
processor or blender. Set aside.

In a large sauté pan over medium to high heat, heat the oil.
Add the onion, Anaheim chile peppers, and garlic. Cook
until the onion is translucent and the peppers are browned
a bit, about 4 to 5 minutes, and transfer to the slow cooker.
Add the remaining ingredients, cover, and cook on low for
8 to 9 hours or on high for 4 to 5 hours, or until beans
are soft.

Serving size: ¾ cup	
Each serving	
Glycemic Index	Low
Glycemic Load	13
Calories	380
Fat	5 g
Saturated Fat	3 g
Carbohydrates	59 g
Fiber	13 g
Protein	26 g

San Francisco–Style Cioppino

Serves 8

3 tablespoons olive oil

1 small fennel bulb, cored and finely chopped (about 1 cup)

1 cup chopped yellow onion

2 large shallots, chopped

½ teaspoon salt

4 large cloves garlic, finely chopped

½ teaspoon red pepper flakes

1 cup dry white wine

2 tablespoons tomato paste

2 (15-ounce) cans diced tomatoes

3 cups low-sodium chicken broth (recipe on page 54)

2 (8-ounce) bottles clam juice

½ teaspoon dried oregano

1 bay leaf

1 pound littleneck clams, scrubbed

1 pound mussels, scrubbed and debearded

1 pound raw large shrimp (26–30 size), peeled and deveined

8 ounces halibut, cut into 2-inch chunks

8 ounces cod, cut into 2-inch chunks

2–3 tablespoons roughly chopped flat-leaf parsley, for garnish

In a large sauté pan over medium heat, heat the oil. Add the fennel, onion, shallots, and salt, and sauté until the onion is translucent, about 4 to 5 minutes. Toss in the garlic and red pepper flakes, and cook for an additional 2 minutes. Transfer the sautéed vegetables from the pan to the slow cooker. Return the pan to the heat and add the wine, making sure to scrape off any bits stuck to the bottom of the pan. Simmer for 2 to 3 minutes and add the tomato paste, canned tomato, chicken broth, clam juice, oregano and bay leaf to the slow cooker. Cover and cook on low for 6 to 8 hours or on high for 3 to 4 hours.

About 30 minutes before serving, put the setting on high, remove the cover, and add the clams, mussels, shrimp, halibut, and cod. Gently stir every 5 minutes. Discard any clams or mussels that do not open. Garnish each serving with fresh chopped parsley.

Serving size: 1 cup	
Each serving	
Glycemic Index	Low
Glycemic Load	1
Calories	358
Fat	11 g
Saturated Fat	2 g
Carbohydrates	15 g
Fiber	2 g
Protein	49 g

Roasted Chanterelle and Leek Soup

Serves 6

1 large leek (about 1 pound), white end washed well, cut in half
  lengthwise and thinly sliced into half moons

1 pound golden chanterelle mushrooms, wiped clean with
  damp paper towel, thinly sliced

3 tablespoons extra virgin olive oil

1 teaspoon salt, divided

1 teaspoon cracked black pepper

2 large bay leaves

4 sprigs fresh thyme

¼ teaspoon black peppercorns

¼ cup chopped white onion

2 large cloves garlic, minced

5 cups low-sodium chicken broth (recipe on page 54)

2 tablespoons chopped fresh flat-leaf parsley

2 tablespoons chopped chives, for garnish

additional extra virgin olive oil or truffle oil, for garnish

Preheat the oven to 400°F. Place the sliced mushrooms and
leek into a large bowl. Drizzle olive oil over the vegetables,
sprinkle with ½ teaspoon salt and ½ teaspoon pepper, and
toss. Place on a baking sheet and roast for 4 to 5 minutes, or
until golden brown. It is okay if they become dark brown, as
they will give the soup flavor.

Place the bay leaves, thyme, and peppercorns on a piece
of cheesecloth, fold, and tie tightly with butcher's twine
to create a sachet. Add the sachet, roasted leeks and
mushrooms, and the onion, garlic, chicken broth, and
parsley to the slow cooker. Cover and cook on low for 5½ to
7 hours or on high for 2½ to 3½ hours. Serve with a chive
garnish and a drizzle of good-quality olive oil or truffle oil.

Serving size: *1 cup*	
Each serving	
Glycemic Index	Low
Glycemic Load	5
Calories	104
Fat	7.3 g
Saturated Fat	1.0 g
Carbohydrates	7.8 g
Fiber	1.5 g
Protein	5 g

Chicken Posole

Serves 6

8 ounces precooked hominy*

4 pounds bone-in chicken drumsticks

2 pounds bone-in chicken breasts, skin removed

½ small white onion, peeled

1 large bay leaf

1 head garlic, unpeeled

1½ teaspoons sea salt, divided

1 teaspoon cracked black pepper, divided

½ teaspoon ground oregano

1 pound tomatillos, peeled and washed

4 cloves garlic

½ cup chopped white onion

2 bunches cilantro

1 serrano chile pepper, deseeded and stem removed

2 quarts (8 cups) low-sodium chicken broth (recipe on page 54), divided

TOPPINGS

1 cup shredded green cabbage

¾ cup thinly sliced radishes

½ cup chopped white onion

6 lime wedges

Place the hominy, chicken, entire half onion, bay leaf, whole garlic head, 1 teaspoon salt, ½ teaspoon pepper and oregano in your slow cooker. In a blender, combine the raw tomatillos, garlic cloves, ½ cup chopped onion, cilantro, serrano chile, ½ teaspoon salt, ½ teaspoon pepper, and 1 cup broth, and blend on high until smooth. Pour the mixture over the chicken in the slow cooker. Add the remaining broth, cover, and cook on low for 8 to 9 hours or on high for 4 to 5 hours, or until the chicken is falling off the bone.

Before serving, remove the chicken and half onion, discard the bones and shred the meat with two forks or with your hands. Put the shredded chicken back into the soup and serve. Garnish each bowl with shredded cabbage, thinly sliced radish, ½ cup chopped onion, and lime wedge.

* Precooked hominy is available at any Hispanic grocery store. If you are unable to find it, use canned hominy.

Serving size: *1 cup*	
Each serving	
Glycemic Index	Low
Glycemic Load	4
Calories	204
Fat	4 g
Saturated Fat	0.7 g
Carbohydrates	26 g
Fiber	5 g
Protein	17 g

Chapter 6

Fish and Poultry

This chapter contains a good variety of chicken dishes, from basic recipes to international ones that will make you feel as if you are cooking gourmet meals. You will also learn to slow cook a whole chicken, as well as different parts of the chicken, such as thighs and breasts. There aren't too many seafood recipes for the slow cooker because fish is very delicate and can easily overcook, but you will discover how to prepare delicious seafood dishes that will leave you asking for more.

Spinach Artichoke Crab Dip

Serves 6

1 cup 1% Greek yogurt

½ cup reduced-fat cream cheese

¼ cup low-fat sour cream

2 (14-ounce) cans artichoke hearts, drained, rinsed, and
  roughly chopped

4 large cloves garlic, finely minced

1 (16-ounce) container frozen chopped spinach, thawed and
  drained very well

½ teaspoon dried parsley

½ teaspoon dried basil

½ teaspoon sea salt

cracked black pepper, to taste

½ cup shredded Parmesan cheese, divided

½ cup shredded part-skim mozzarella cheese, divided

8 ounces fresh crab meat, finely pulled and checked for
  cartilage

In a large mixing bowl, combine the yogurt, cream cheese,
and sour cream, and whisk until the cream cheese is evenly
incorporated. Add the artichoke hearts, garlic, spinach,
parsley, basil, salt, pepper and ¼ cup each of the Parmesan
and mozzarella cheeses. Fold in the crab meat using a
rubber spatula. Transfer the mixture to the slow cooker
and spread it out evenly with the spatula. Top with the
remaining ¼ cup each of the Parmesan and mozzarella.
Cover and cook on high for 1 to 1½ hours, or on low for 2
to 2½ hours, or until the cheeses on top have completely
melted and the dip is heated through.

Serving size: ½ cup	
Each serving	
Glycemic Index	Low
Glycemic Load	2
Calories	274
Fat	14 g
Saturated Fat	8 g
Carbohydrates	13 g
Fiber	4 g
Protein	25 g

Spicy Almond Chicken
Serves 4

¼ cup almond meal

½ teaspoons cracked black pepper

4 (4-ounce) boneless, skinless chicken breasts, fat trimmed

2 tablespoons melted coconut oil, divided

2 tablespoons chili paste, such as Sambal

2 tablespoons coconut vinegar or rice wine vinegar

¼ cup water

1 large clove garlic, minced

½ inch fresh ginger, peeled and minced

¼ teaspoon red pepper flakes

½ cup sliced almonds, toasted

Combine the almond meal and cracked black pepper in a large Ziploc bag. Add the chicken and shake to coat. Heat 1 tablespoon coconut oil in a large skillet over medium heat. Brown the chicken about 1 minute on each side, then transfer to the slow cooker. In a small bowl, whisk together the remaining 1 tablespoon coconut oil with the chili paste, coconut vinegar, water, garlic, ginger, and red pepper flakes. Pour the sauce over the chicken, cover, and cook on low for 2 to 3 hours. Top the cooked chicken with the toasted almonds and serve.

Serving size: *4 ounces*	
Each serving	
Glycemic Index	Very Low
Glycemic Load	1
Calories	223
Fat	17 g
Saturated Fat	7 g
Carbohydrates	7 g
Fiber	2 g
Protein	12 g

Herbed Whole Chicken
Serves 4

1 cup chopped white onion

4 large cloves garlic, finely chopped

1 tablespoon minced rosemary

1 teaspoon minced fresh thyme

1 teaspoon minced fresh oregano

1 teaspoon paprika

1 teaspoon lemon zest

2 teaspoons sea salt

1 teaspoon cracked black pepper

1 (3- to 4-pound) chicken, giblets removed

Place the chopped onion in the bottom of the slow cooker. Combine the garlic, rosemary, thyme, oregano, paprika, lemon zest, salt, and pepper, and rub them on the chicken with your hands, making sure to lift the skin on the breast and rub the mixture on the meat under the skin, as well. Cook on low for 7 to 8 hours, or on high for 3½ to 4 hours, or until the chicken is falling off the bone. Save the juices to make a delicious sauce or chicken broth.

Serving size: *3 ounces light or dark meat, no skin*	
Each serving	
Glycemic Index	Low
Glycemic Load	0
Calories	101; 107
Fat	1 g; 3 g
Saturated Fat	0 g; 0 g
Carbohydrates	2 g; 2 g
Fiber	0.2 g; 0.2 g
Protein	18 g; 18 g

Mustard Balsamic Glazed Chicken with Butternut Squash

Serves 4

1 teaspoon stoneground mustard

¼ cup balsamic vinegar

¼ cup extra virgin olive oil

½ teaspoon chopped fresh thyme

½ teaspoon sea salt

cracked black pepper, to taste

12 ounces boneless, skinless chicken breasts, fat trimmed and
  cut into 1-inch pieces

½ pound butternut squash, peeled, halved, and seeded

In a small bowl, whisk together the mustard, balsamic vinegar, olive oil, thyme, salt, and pepper to taste. Place the chicken into a large Ziploc bag and add the mustard mixture, working the marinade into the chicken with your fingers on the outside of the sealed bag. Refrigerate overnight or for at least 30 minutes.

With a mandolin or knife, cut the butternut squash into paper-thin slices, less than ¼ inch thick. Line the bottom of the slow cooker with the squash slices. Pour the chicken and marinade on top of the squash. Cover and cook on low for 3 to 4 hours or on high for 1 to 1½ hours, or until the squash is tender when pierced with a fork. Drizzle the chicken and squash with sauce from the slow cooker when serving.

Serving size: *3 ounces chicken, ¼ cup butternut squash*	
Each serving	
Glycemic Index	Medium
Glycemic Load	3
Calories	189
Fat	10 g
Saturated Fat	2 g
Carbohydrates	7 g
Fiber	2 g
Protein	20 g

Tandoori Chicken
Serves 4

TANDOORI MARINADE

2½ cups nonfat plain Greek yogurt, divided

2 large cloves garlic, minced

1 teaspoon minced fresh ginger

2 tablespoons fresh lemon juice

1 teaspoon ground cumin

1 teaspoon paprika plus ½ teaspoon, divided

½ teaspoon ground coriander plus ½ teaspoon, divided

¼ teaspoon ground cardamom plus ¼ teaspoon, divided

½ teaspoon cayenne plus ½ teaspoon, divided

½ teaspoon ground cinnamon plus ½ teaspoon, divided

½ teaspoon sea salt

CHICKEN

12 ounces boneless, skinless chicken breasts, fat trimmed and
  cut into 1-inch pieces

1 (15-ounce) can garbanzo beans, drained and rinsed

1 cup chopped fresh tomato

In a large bowl, combine 1 cup Greek yogurt and the rest
of the marinade ingredients, reserving the second batch
of spices in a separate small bowl for later use. Taste the
marinade and season with additional salt if necessary. Add
the chicken to the bowl with the marinade, and mix until
the chicken is evenly coated. Cover the bowl, place in the
refrigerator, and marinate overnight or for at least 1 hour.

Place the garbanzo beans and chopped tomato in the
bottom of the slow cooker, and set the marinated chicken
on top. Cover and cook on low for 4 to 4½ hours or on
high for 2 to 2½ hours, or until the chicken is tender. Add
the remaining 1½ cups yogurt and reserved spices to the

chickpea and chicken mixture, and stir well. Place lid back on, cook on high for an additional 15 to 20 minutes, or until heated through.

Serving Suggestion: Serve with fresh cilantro and lime wedges as garnish.

Serving size: *3 ounces chicken, ¼ cup garbanzo beans with sauce*	
Each serving	
Glycemic Index	Low
Glycemic Load	11
Calories	314
Fat	4 g
Saturated Fat	0.8 g
Carbohydrates	35 g
Fiber	6 g
Protein	35 g

Chicken Fajita Wraps

Serves 4

12 ounces boneless, skinless chicken breast, cut into long, thin strips

3 tablespoons fresh lime juice

1 teaspoon dried oregano

1½ teaspoon chili powder

2 teaspoons paprika

½ teaspoon ground cumin

½ teaspoon cayenne

¼ teaspoon garlic powder

½ teaspoon sea salt

½ teaspoon cracked black pepper

½ large onion, cut into ¼-inch-thick slices

1 cup sliced green bell pepper, ¼-inch-thick,

1 cup sliced yellow bell pepper, ¼-inch-thick

1 cup sliced orange bell pepper, ¼-inch-thick

1 cup sliced red bell pepper, ¼-inch-thick

4 (7-inch) whole wheat tortillas

1 cup shredded romaine

½ large avocado, pit removed, meat scooped out and lightly mashed

⅓ cup 2% Greek yogurt

Combine the chicken, lime juice, oregano, chili powder, paprika, cumin, cayenne, garlic powder, salt, and black pepper in a large Ziploc bag. Marinate overnight or at least 30 minutes, Place the onion and bell peppers in the slow cooker. Place the marinated chicken on top of the vegetables in the slow cooker, along with any juices in the bag. Cover and cook on low for 3 to 4 hours or on high for 1 to 1½ hours, or until chicken is tender. Scoop cooked chicken and vegetables into the center of each tortilla into a vertical line. Top with ¼ cup shredded romaine, ¼ of the mashed avocado and a dollop of Greek yogurt. Fold the left side of the tortilla over the chicken and vegetables, fold the bottom of the tortilla upwards and tuck in under the fold. Continue rolling until completely wrapped. Repeat with remaining tortillas.

Serving Suggestion: Be creative with your toppings for the chicken and vegetables. Serve with your favorite fresh salsa, shredded low-fat cheese, or a serving of black beans.

Serving size: *1 wrap with 3 ounces chicken breast, 1 cup vegetables, 2 tablespoons avocado and 1 tablespoon Greek yogurt*	
Each serving	
Glycemic Index	Low
Glycemic Load	4
Calories	348
Fat	14 g
Saturated Fat	2 g
Carbohydrates	32 g
Fiber	13 g
Protein	32 g

Red Enchilada Sauce

Makes 8 cups

3 large dried pasilla or ancho chile peppers, seeds and stems
   removed

5 dried chiles de arbol, stems snapped off

¼ teaspoon cumin seeds

1 cup chopped onion

2 large cloves garlic

3 (15-ounce) cans whole peeled tomatoes

½ teaspoon sea salt

Heat a large dry skillet on high heat. Add both types of
chile peppers to the hot pan, stirring every 10 seconds
or so. Continue cooking until the chiles blacken and
are fragrant. Remove from the heat and add to the slow
cooker. Add the cumin seeds to the same pan and, stirring
constantly, toast until fragrant, about 30 seconds.

Place the toasted cumin and the remaining ingredients in
the slow cooker, and mix well. Cover and cook on high for
1 to 1½ hours, or until the onions are soft. Transfer the
mixture to a blender, and blend until smooth. Taste and
season with additional salt to your liking. If you like your
sauce thinner, strain through a fine-mesh strainer if you
have one; otherwise any strainer will do.

Chef's Tip: If you make a large batch of sauce, freeze half of
it in an airtight container for future use.

Serving size: *1 cup*	
Each serving	
Glycemic Index	Low
Glycemic Load	1
Calories	37
Fat	0.3 g
Saturated Fat	0 g
Carbohydrates	8.5 g
Fiber	2 g
Protein	2 g

Chicken Enchilada Casserole

Serves 4

1 pound boneless, skinless chicken breasts, fat trimmed

8 (6-inch) corn tortillas

1 large zucchini, shredded and squeezed between paper towels
  to drain liquid

2 cups shredded cheddar cheese, divided

½ teaspoon ground cumin

½ teaspoon sea salt

cracked black pepper, to taste

4 cups red enchilada sauce (recipe on page 98), divided

¼ cup thinly sliced green onion, white parts discarded

Bring a large pot of water to a boil. Cut the chicken breasts
in half and add to the boiling water. Boil for 10 to 12
minutes, or until the chicken pulls apart with two forks and
is no longer pink in the center. Remove the chicken from
the water and let cool at room temperature. Use two forks
or your fingers to pull the meat apart into thin pieces. (If
you are pressed for time, use a precooked rotisserie chicken
and pull the meat from it.)

Heat a large dry skillet over high heat. Once the pan is
hot, add the tortillas individually and warm each slightly
on both sides. Place the warmed tortillas in a stack inside
a folded kitchen towel to keep warm and set aside. In a
medium bowl, combine the cooked, shredded chicken,
drained zucchini, 1 cup cheese, cumin, salt, and pepper.
Spread 2 cups enchilada sauce in the bottom of the slow
cooker. Scoop ½ cup of the chicken and cheese mixture
into the middle of a warmed tortilla. Roll the tortilla up
and place seam side down on top of the sauce. Repeat until
you have filled all the tortillas and placed them in the slow

cooker. Top the rolled tortillas with the remaining 2 cups enchilada sauce and 1 cup cheese. Cover and cook on low for 3 to 3½ hours or on high for 1½ to 2 hours. Garnish with the green onion and serve casserole style.

Serving size: *2 corn tortillas, 4 ounces chicken, ¼ cup enchilada sauce*	
Each serving	
Glycemic Index	Low
Glycemic Load	16
Calories	434
Fat	22 g
Saturated Fat	12 g
Carbohydrates	38 g
Fiber	3 g
Protein	22 g

Turkey and Veggie Stuffed Acorn Squash

Serves 2

1 medium acorn squash, about 4 inches in diameter

2 teaspoons sea salt, divided

1 teaspoon cracked black pepper, divided

1 tablespoon extra virgin olive oil

1 small carrot, chopped (about ½ cup)

¼ cup chopped white onion

8 ounces lean ground turkey

1 large clove garlic, minced

1 teaspoon paprika

½ teaspoon dried oregano

2 large tomatoes, grated, about 1 cup pulp

½ cup low-sodium vegetable broth (recipe on page 56)

Cut the acorn squash in half, scoop out the seeds, and season the inside with ½ teaspoon salt and ½ teaspoon pepper. Heat the olive oil in a medium sauté pan over medium heat. Add the carrot and onion, and cook for 4 to 5 minutes before adding the ground turkey. Break up any large pieces of turkey with a spatula or fork, and cook until the turkey begins to brown, about 7 to 8 minutes. Add the garlic, paprika, and oregano, and continue cooking for 2 to 3 minutes. Then add the grated tomato, vegetable broth and the remaining salt, and pepper. Stir until the tomato pulp heats, about 1 minute, and remove the pan from the heat.

Evenly scoop the turkey mixture into each acorn squash half. Pour in enough water to cover the bottom of the slow cooker, between ½ and ¾ cup, and carefully set the acorn squash halves in the cooker. Cover and cook on low for 7 to

8 hours or on high for 3½ to 4 hours, or until the squash is tender and the inside is easily pierced with a fork.

Serving size: ½ squash with 1 cup turkey and vegetable mixture	
Each serving	
Glycemic Index	High
Glycemic Load	10
Calories	344
Fat	16 g
Saturated Fat	4 g
Carbohydrates	31 g
Fiber	5 g
Protein	25 g

Almond Sauce Chicken

Serves 4

1 cup whole almonds

1½ cups roughly chopped tomato

½ cup chopped white onion

1 large clove garlic, roughly chopped

1 teaspoon jalapeño pepper, roughly chopped, deseeded if less
  heat is desired

¼ cup packed cilantro

½ slice toasted sprouted grain bread, torn into pieces

1½ cups low-sodium chicken broth (recipe on page 54)

2 tablespoons fresh lime juice

1 teaspoon sea salt

½ teaspoon cracked black pepper

4 (3-ounce) boneless, skinless chicken breasts

Toast the almonds: Heat a large dry skillet over high heat,
and add the almonds when the pan is hot. Shake the pan
often until the almonds start to brown and become fragrant,
about 2 to 3 minutes. Remove and set aside.

In the same pan on high heat, add the tomato, onion,
garlic, and jalapeño. Toast them until they blacken, moving
them with a spatula every 3 to 4 minutes. Turn the heat off
and combine the toasted almonds, blackened vegetables,
cilantro, toasted bread, broth, and lime juice in a blender.
Pulse and then blend on high speed until the sauce is
smooth. Season the sauce with salt and pepper.

Spray the inside of your slow cooker with nonstick spray
and lay the chicken breasts in an even layer. Spread the
sauce to completely cover the chicken. Cover and cook

on low for 2½ to 3 hours or on high for 1 to ½ hours,
or until chicken is no longer pink in the center and easily
pulls apart.

Serving size: *3 ounces chicken, 3 tablespoons sauce*	
Each serving	
Glycemic Index	Low
Glycemic Load	2
Calories	346
Fat	21 g
Saturated Fat	2 g
Carbohydrates	14 g
Fiber	6 g
Protein	29 g

Duck Legs with Baby Bok Choy and Shiitake Mushrooms

Serves 2

1½ pounds baby bok choy, halved

1½ cups thinly sliced shiitake mushrooms

2 tablespoons extra virgin olive oil

2 (4-ounce) duck legs

¼ teaspoon Chinese five-spice powder

1 teaspoon sea salt

½ teaspoon cracked black pepper

3 tablespoons soy sauce

⅛ teaspoon red pepper flakes

Line the bottom of your slow cooker with the halved baby bok choy. Top with the sliced mushrooms. Heat a large sauté pan over high heat. Once the pan is hot, add the oil. Meanwhile, season both sides of each duck leg with the Chinese five-spice powder, salt, and pepper, and sear for 1 to 2 minutes on each side, until the meat is dark brown and makes a nice crust. Remove the legs from the pan and place on top of the vegetables in the slow cooker. Add the soy sauce and red pepper flakes. Cover and cook on low for 5 to 6 hours or on high for 3 to 3½ hours, or until the duck meat is fully cooked and falling off the bone.

Serving size: *1 duck leg, ¾ cup vegetables*	
Each serving	
Glycemic Index	Low
Glycemic Load	1
Calories	410
Fat	27 g
Saturated Fat	5 g
Carbohydrates	8 g
Fiber	1 g
Protein	38 g

Chicken Tagine with Artichokes and Peas

Serves 4

1 tablespoon extra virgin olive oil

1 medium onion, chopped

3 large cloves garlic, minced

1 (14-ounce) can artichoke hearts, drained, rinsed, and
  quartered

8 ounces boneless, skinless chicken breasts, fat trimmed and
  cut into 1-inch pieces

8 ounces boneless, skinless chicken thigh, cut into 1-inch
  pieces

1 teaspoon sea salt

½ teaspoon cracked black pepper

½ teaspoon ground ginger

¼ teaspoon ground cumin

½ teaspoon turmeric

¼ teaspoon ground allspice

Pinch of crumbled saffron threads

2 cups chopped fresh tomato

1 cup frozen English peas

zest of 1 lemon

In a large sauté pan over medium to high heat, heat the
oil. Add the onion and garlic, and cook until the onion is
translucent, 2 to 3 minutes. Line the bottom of your slow
cooker with the artichoke hearts, then top with the sautéed
onion and garlic. In a large bowl, combine the chicken
with the salt, pepper, ginger, cumin, turmeric, allspice, and
saffron, and mix to coat well. Spread the chicken on top
of the artichoke hearts, onion, and garlic, and top with the
tomato, peas, and lemon zest. Cover and cook on low for

8 to 9 hours or on high for 4 to 4½ hours, or until chicken
is tender.

Serving size: 3 ounces chicken, 1 cup vegetables	
Each serving	
Glycemic Index	Low
Glycemic Load	3
Calories	261
Fat	7 g
Saturated Fat	1 g
Carbohydrates	26 g
Fiber	11 g
Protein	25 g

Spiced Sockeye Salmon with Greens

Serves 4

1 tablespoon extra virgin olive oil

2 cups thinly sliced yellow onion

1 bunch Swiss chard, roughly chopped (about 4 cups)

1 tablespoon red wine vinegar

½ cup low-sodium chicken broth (recipe on page 54)

¼ teaspoon turmeric

¼ teaspoon cayenne

⅛ teaspoon ground cumin

⅛ teaspoon garlic powder

¾ teaspoon sea salt

½ teaspoon cracked black pepper

4 (3-ounce) sockeye salmon fillets

1 large lemon, cut into 4 wedges

In a small sauté pan over medium to high heat, heat the oil. Add the onion, and cook for 4 to 5 minutes, or until softened. Transfer to the slow cooker and top with the Swiss chard. Drizzle the red wine vinegar and broth over the greens.

In a small bowl, combine the turmeric, cayenne, cumin, garlic powder, salt, and pepper, and whisk or mix with a fork. Using your hands, rub the spice mixture all over the salmon, and place on top of the chard, making sure to leave at least ½ inch between fillets. Cover and cook on low for 1 to 1½ hours, or until the salmon is tender and easily flakes with a fork. Right before serving, squeeze the juice of 1 lemon wedge over the top of each fillet.

Serving size: *3 ounces fish, 1 cup vegetables*	
Each serving	
Glycemic Index	Low
Glycemic Load	1
Calories	319
Fat	13 g
Saturated Fat	2 g
Carbohydrates	19 g
Fiber	7 g
Protein	34 g

Tropical Mahi Mahi with Mango Jalapeño Salsa
Serves 4

MAHI MAHI

1 bunch green onions, root ends cut off

4 (3-ounce) mahi mahi fish fillets

½ teaspoon sea salt

½ teaspoon cracked black pepper

½ teaspoon paprika

¼ teaspoon ground cumin

zest of 1 lime

4 tablespoons fresh lime juice

MANGO JALAPEÑO SALSA

½ cup finely diced mango

½ cup chopped tomato

¼ cup chopped red onion

1 teaspoon minced jalapeño pepper

2 tablespoon chopped cilantro

1 tablespoon fresh lime juice

¼ teaspoon sea salt

Cover the bottom of the slow cooker with the green onions. Season the mahi mahi with the salt, pepper, paprika, cumin, and lime zest. Place the seasoned fillets in the slow cooker, leaving at least ½ inch between fillets, and drizzle 1 tablespoon lime juice over each one. Cover and cook on low for 1½ to 2 hours, or until the fish easily flakes with a fork.

While the fish cooks, make the salsa by mixing together the mango, tomato, red onion, jalapeño, cilantro, 1 tablespoon lime juice, and salt. Discard the green onions, and serve the fillets with 1 tablespoon of the salsa over each.

Serving size: *3 ounces fish, 1 tablespoon salsa*	
Each serving	
Glycemic Index	Low
Glycemic Load	1
Calories	147
Fat	1 g
Saturated Fat	0 g
Carbohydrates	16 g
Fiber	2 g
Protein	21 g

Swordfish Casserole

Serves 4

12 ounces swordfish, skinless, cut into 1-inch cubes

1 teaspoon sea salt

½ teaspoon crack black pepper

2 cups finely chopped celery

1 large red bell pepper, finely chopped (about 1½ cups)

1 cup finely chopped yellow onion

3 cups finely chopped fresh tomato

½ cup loosely packed de-stemmed dill

2 tablespoons capers

Season the swordfish with salt and pepper. Place the celery and bell pepper and then the onion in the slow cooker. Distribute the swordfish cubes on top. Then place the tomato, dill, and capers over the fish. Cover and cook on low for 4 to 4½ hours or on high for 2 to 2½ hours, or until the fish is fully cooked and flaky. Leave the lid on for 30 minutes after turning off the slow cooker.

Serving size: *3 ounces fish, 1 cup vegetables*	
Each serving	
Glycemic Index	Low
Glycemic Load	1
Calories	201
Fat	5 g
Saturated Fat	1 g
Carbohydrates	16 g
Fiber	4 g
Protein	24 g

Chapter 7

Red Meat and Pork

Red meat is the perfect candidate for slow cooking. Not only does it have a lot of flavor, but you can use many different cuts of beef, even inexpensive cuts that are usually tough when you cook them on the stovetop. The great thing about using inexpensive cuts of beef is that you can slow cook them and they will come out extremely tender. Pork chops and pork loin are leaner than other cuts of pork and can easily overcook, so keep a close eye on them when you reach the minimum recommended cooking time. Larger pieces of pork, such as pork shoulder, are fantastic candidates for a slow cooker as well. Avoid overnight braising in the oven by using the slow cooker to cook your meat, and your results will be just as good, if not better.

Tender Pork Loin and Nectarines

Serves 4

2 large cloves garlic, minced

1 teaspoon sea salt

½ teaspoon cracked black pepper

1 tablespoon chopped thyme

¾ pound center cut boneless pork tenderloin

1½ cups halved and thinly sliced red onion

½ cup low-sodium chicken broth (recipe on page 54)

2 cups nectarines, pit removed, thinly sliced

2 tablespoons sherry vinegar

In a small bowl, combine the garlic, salt, pepper and thyme. Using your hands, rub the seasoning all over the pork loin. Wrap the loin in plastic wrap and place in the refrigerator overnight or for at least 30 minutes. Line the bottom of your slow cooker with the red onion slices and pour in the chicken broth. Place the pork on top of the onion, and then top the pork with the nectarines. Drizzle the sherry vinegar over the top. Cover and cook on low for 4½ to 5 hours or until tender and pork is no longer pink in the center.

Serving size: 3 ounces pork; ½ cup nectarines	
Each serving	
Glycemic Index	Low
Glycemic Load	3
Calories	166
Fat	3 g
Saturated Fat	0 g
Carbohydrates	13 g
Fiber	2 g
Protein	20 g

Classic Pork Chops and Apples

Serves 4

½ cup very thinly sliced red onion

4 (3-ounce) boneless pork loin chops

½ teaspoon sea salt

½ teaspoon cracked black pepper

3 tablespoons Worcestershire sauce

¼ cup cider vinegar

2 large Granny Smith apples, peeled and thinly sliced

½ teaspoon ground cinnamon

¼ teaspoon ground ginger

Spread the onion slices in an even layer on the bottom of your slow cooker. Pat the pork dry with a paper towel, and season with the salt and pepper. Place the chops on top of the onion, being careful not to overlap them too much. In a small bowl, whisk the Worcestershire sauce and cider vinegar, and pour the mixture over the chops. In a medium bowl, toss the apples slices with the cinnamon and ginger, and place them on top of the chops. Cover and cook on low for 4 to 4½ hours or on high for 2 to 2½ hours, or until pork chops are no longer pink in the center.

Serving size: *3 ounces pork, ½ cup apples and onions*	
Each serving	
Glycemic Index	Low
Glycemic Load	4
Calories	224
Fat	9 g
Saturated Fat	3 g
Carbohydrates	17 g
Fiber	3 g
Protein	18 g

Pulled Pork Tacos with Tangy Coleslaw

Serves 8

COLESLAW

2 cups shredded red cabbage

2 cups shredded green cabbage

1½ cups shredded carrot (about 2 large carrots)

½ cup apple cider vinegar

1 teaspoon sea salt

½ teaspoon cracked black pepper

PULLED PORK TACOS

2 tablespoons coconut palm sugar

1 tablespoon paprika

1 teaspoon dry mustard

½ teaspoon cayenne

1 teaspoon sea salt

½ teaspoon cracked black pepper

1 (2-pound) pork shoulder, bone-in, fat trimmed

⅓ cup brown mustard

½ cup low-sodium chicken broth (recipe on page 54)

½ cup apple cider vinegar

2 teaspoons Worcestershire sauce

1 tablespoon chopped canned chipotles in adobo sauce

½ teaspoon red pepper flakes

16 (6-inch) corn tortillas

To make the coleslaw, mix together all the coleslaw ingredients in a large bowl. Place in the refrigerator for at least 30 minutes to let the flavors meld and the cabbage pickle.

To prepare the pork, thoroughly combine the sugar, paprika, dry mustard, cayenne, salt, and pepper in a small bowl. Using your hands, rub the spice mixture all over the pork. Place in a Ziploc bag or covered on a plate and refrigerate overnight or let sit for 1 hour at room temperature. In a medium bowl, whisk together the brown mustard, chicken broth, vinegar, Worcestershire sauce, adobo peppers, and red pepper flakes. Place the seasoned pork in the slow cooker, and pour the liquid mixture over it.

Cover and cook on low for 8 to 9 hours, or until the pork is very tender and easily shreds. Pull the meat into strands using two forks. Warm the tortillas individually in a skillet over medium heat, scoop ½ cup pulled pork onto each tortilla, and top with coleslaw.

Serving size: 4 ounces pork, 2 tortillas, 1 cup coleslaw	
Each serving	
Glycemic Index	Low
Glycemic Load	15
Calories	462
Fat	25 g
Saturated Fat	9 g
Carbohydrates	38 g
Fiber	5 g
Protein	23 g

Lamb-Stuffed Bell Peppers

Serves 4

12 ounces ground lamb

¼ cup uncooked brown rice

1 (28-ounce) can diced tomatoes

½ cup chopped white onion

2 large cloves garlic, minced

½ cup chopped celery

2 tablespoons chopped mint

2 tablespoons chopped parsley

½ teaspoon ground cinnamon

1 teaspoon sea salt

½ teaspoon cracked black pepper

4 large bell peppers, assorted colors

In a large bowl, mix together the lamb, rice, tomatoes, onion, garlic, celery, mint, parsley, cinnamon, salt, and pepper by hand. Slice off the tops of the bell peppers and set aside. Remove the seeds and ribs from the peppers, and rinse under running water to wash out any seeds. Pat dry. Stuff each pepper with equal amounts of the lamb mixture.

Set the stuffed peppers in your slow cooker and put the tops back on. Pour water around the base of the peppers, using only enough to cover the bottom of the slow cooker. Cover and cook on low for about 5 to 6 hours or on high for 2½ to 3 hours, or until the rice in the lamb mixture is fully cooked.

Serving size: *1 bell pepper, ¾ cup stuffing*	
Each serving	
Glycemic Index	Low
Glycemic Load	7
Calories	276
Fat	14 g
Saturated Fat	6 g
Carbohydrates	22 g
Fiber	4 g
Protein	13 g

Herbed Pork Chops

Serves 4

1 pound zucchini, cut into ¼-inch slices

½ chopped small white onion (about ½ cup)

4 (3-ounce) boneless pork chops

1 tablespoon extra virgin olive oil

½ teaspoon sea salt

½ teaspoon cracked black pepper

3 tablespoons chopped fresh rosemary

2 tablespoons chopped fresh sage

1 teaspoon lemon zest

1 large clove garlic, finely minced

Pat the pork chops dry with paper towels. Combine the olive oil, salt, pepper, rosemary, sage, lemon zest, and garlic in a small bowl, and mix well. Using your hands, rub the herb mixture all over each pork chop. Place in a Ziploc bag or covered on a plate and refrigerate overnight or let sit for 1 hour at room temperature. Spread the zucchini and onion in an even layer on the bottom of your slow cooker. Arrange the chops on top of the vegetables. Cover and cook on low for 8 to 8½ hours or on high for 4 to 4½ hours, or until the chops are tender.

Serving size: *3 ounces pork, ¾ cup vegetables*	
Each serving	
Glycemic Index	Low
Glycemic Load	2
Calories	217
Fat	13 g
Saturated Fat	4 g
Carbohydrates	7 g
Fiber	3 g
Protein	18 g

Polish Sausage and Cabbage

Serves 4

1 tablespoon caraway seeds

1 medium green cabbage, cut into quarters and cored
   (about 2 pounds)

2 large cloves garlic, minced

½ teaspoon sea salt

½ teaspoon cracked black pepper

12 ounces Polish pork sausages

2 cups low-sodium chicken broth (recipe on page 54)

Toast the caraway seeds: Heat a small sauté pan over high heat, and add the caraway seeds when the pan is hot. Stirring often, toast the seeds until fragrant, about 2 to 3 minutes. Place the toasted seeds in a spice grinder or blender and pulse once, to gently crush them. Set aside.

Place the sectioned cabbage in the bottom of your slow cooker, and sprinkle the garlic and toasted caraway seeds on top. Season with salt and pepper. Place the Polish sausage on top of the cabbage and pour broth over the sausage, cover, and cook on low for 10 to 11 hours or on high for 5 to 6 hours.

Serving size: *3 ounces sausage, 1 cup cabbage*	
Each serving	
Glycemic Index	Low
Glycemic Load	1
Calories	362
Fat	25 g
Saturated Fat	9 g
Carbohydrates	19 g
Fiber	7 g
Protein	18 g

Traditional Bolognese Sauce

Serves 4

2 tablespoons extra virgin olive oil

8 ounces ground beef chuck

8 ounces ground pork

1 (28-ounce) can whole peeled tomatoes

1 large carrot, finely chopped

1 medium onion, chopped

1 celery stalk, chopped

2 large cloves garlic, minced

¼ cup tomato paste

¼ cup red wine

1 teaspoon finely chopped fresh oregano

1 teaspoon finely chopped fresh thyme

2 bay leaves

1 teaspoon sea salt

½ teaspoon cracked black pepper

Heat a large sauté pan over medium heat. Once the pan is hot, add the oil and then the ground beef and ground pork, making sure to break up any large lumps with a spatula. Once the meat has browned, about 4 to 5 minutes, drain the fat from the pan. Place the browned meat in your slow cooker, add the remaining ingredients, and mix well. Cover and cook on low for 7 to 9 hours or on high for 4 to 5 hours.

Serving Suggestion: This sauce is great on pasta, can be used for lasagna, served with meatballs, or any meat of your choice.

Serving size: ½ cup	
Each serving	
Glycemic Index	Low
Glycemic Load	5
Calories	315
Fat	19 g
Saturated Fat	6 g
Carbohydrates	20 g
Fiber	5 g
Protein	16 g

Braised Beef Short Ribs
Serves 4

1 tablespoon extra virgin olive oil

1 tablespoon mustard seeds

½ cup balsamic vinegar

½ cup low-sodium beef broth (recipe on page 58)

3 tablespoons soy sauce

2 large cloves garlic, crushed

½ teaspoon red pepper flakes

¼ teaspoon cracked black pepper

3 pounds beef short ribs, fat trimmed to ⅛ inch*

1 large yellow onion, halved and thinly sliced (about 3 cups)

Heat the oil in a small pan on medium heat. Once the oil is hot, add the mustard seeds, stirring often. Place a loosely fitting lid or spatter screen over the pan, as the seeds tend to pop. After 2 to 3 minutes, when they have browned, remove them from the heat.

Combine the balsamic vinegar, beef broth, soy sauce, garlic, red pepper flakes, mustard seeds and oil, and black pepper in a medium bowl, and whisk well. Pour the mixture into a large Ziploc bag, add the short ribs, and seal tightly, pushing as much air out of the bag as you can. Marinate in the refrigerator overnight or for at least 1 hour.

Place the onion in the bottom of your slow cooker, then lay the marinated shorts ribs on top of the onion, placing them on their sides if they are too large to fit in a single layer. Drizzle the marinade over the ribs, cover, and cook on low for 10 to 12 hours or on high for 5 to 6 hours, or until the rib meat is falling off the bone.

* Usually, 2 small short ribs per person should suffice, but use your discretion, as bone density will affect the final weight. Short ribs usually are very fatty and will leave a greasy cap on top of any juices in the slow cooker. That's why it's important to trim the fat before cooking. Alternatively, you can broil the marinated short ribs in the oven for about 5 minutes and then drain them on paper towels before placing them in the slow cooker.

Serving size: *2 (6-ounce) ribs with bone, or 4-ounce rib meat (fat and caloric content may vary depending on how much fat is trimmed prior to cooking)*

Each serving	
Glycemic Index	Low
Glycemic Load	1
Calories	255
Fat	12 g
Saturated Fat	5 g
Carbohydrates	13 g
Fiber	2 g
Protein	24 g

Asian-Style Skirt Steak

Serves 4

3 tablespoons soy sauce

1 tablespoon rice wine vinegar

¼ cup hoisin

1 inch fresh ginger, peeled and finely minced, or 1 teaspoon
  ground ginger

2 large cloves garlic, minced

¼ teaspoon red pepper flakes

¾ pound skirt steak, fat trimmed and membrane removed

2 stalks lemongrass, outer leaves peeled, cut into 2-inch pieces

2 cups red bell pepper, chopped into 1-inch pieces

½ cup low-sodium beef broth (recipe on page 58)

4 tablespoons chopped green onion, green part only

In a small bowl, combine the soy sauce, vinegar, hoisin,
ginger, garlic, and red pepper flakes, and mix well. Place the
skirt steak in a large Ziploc bag or a shallow pan. Add the
marinade, seal the bag or cover the pan, and marinate in the
refrigerator overnight or for at least 1 hour.

Lay the lemongrass in the bottom of your slow cooker.
Place the bell pepper on top, then the steak, and finally the
marinade and the beef broth. Cover and cook on low for
5½ to 6 hours or on high for 2½ to 3 hours, or until meat
is very tender and easily pulls apart. Garnish meat with
chopped green onion.

Serving size: *3 ounces steak, 1 cup vegetables*	
Each serving	
Glycemic Index	Low
Glycemic Load	3
Calories	254
Fat	11 g
Saturated Fat	4 g
Carbohydrates	14 g
Fiber	1 g
Protein	25 g

Lamb and Olive Tagine

Serves 4

1 large yellow onion, ½ thinly sliced, ½ chopped

1 pound lamb shoulder, fat trimmed, meat cut into
  2-inch cubes

1 tablespoon minced fresh ginger

¼ cup packed chopped cilantro

½ teaspoon lemon zest

3 tablespoons fresh lemon juice

1 teaspoon turmeric

1 teaspoon paprika

1 teaspoon crumbled saffron threads

½ teaspoon ground cloves

¼ cup chopped fresh tarragon

1 tablespoon tomato paste

¾ teaspoon sea salt

½ teaspoon cracked black pepper

¾ cup low-sodium beef broth (recipe on page 58)

1 cup green olives with pits, drained and rinsed if in brine

Place the sliced onion in a single layer in the bottom of your
slow cooker. In a large bowl, mix the cubes of lamb with the
chopped onion, ginger, cilantro, lemon zest, lemon juice,
turmeric, paprika, saffron, cloves, tarragon, tomato paste,
salt, and pepper, and add the mixture to the slow cooker,
along with the broth and olives. Cover and cook on low for
7 to 8 hours or on high for 4 to 5 hours, or until the lamb is
very tender.

Serving size: ¾ cup lamb and olive mixture	
Each serving	
Glycemic Index	Low
Glycemic Load	2
Calories	480
Fat	36 g
Saturated Fat	12 g
Carbohydrates	17 g
Fiber	2 g
Protein	22 g

Round Roast with Pearl Onions

Serves 8

1 teaspoon sea salt

½ teaspoon freshly ground pepper

1 teaspoon minced fresh rosemary

½ teaspoon lemon zest

4 large cloves garlic, minced

1 tablespoon onion powder

1 teaspoon Dijon mustard

1½ teaspoons brown sugar

1½ pounds beef round roast, fat trimmed

2 tablespoons grapeseed oil

1 pound pearl onions, peeled

¼ cup low-sodium beef broth (recipe on page 58)

1 tablespoon cornstarch

1½ tablespoons water

In a small bowl, mix together the salt, pepper, rosemary, lemon zest, garlic, onion powder, mustard and brown sugar. Using your hands, rub this mixture all over the roast. In a large sauté pan, heat the grapeseed oil until very hot. Place the roast in the hot pan and sear all sides evenly, about 30 seconds per side. Place the pearl onions in the bottom of the slow cooker, and set the roast on top. Pour in the broth, cover, and cook on low for 6 to 7 hours, or until internal temperature of the meat reaches at least 140 degrees.

Remove the roast and place it on a platter to rest for at least 10 minutes before slicing. Scoop the pearl onions out with a slotted spoon. Pour the beef liquid into a small pot and bring to a boil. In a small bowl, whisk the cornstarch with the water and pour the mixture into the boiling beef liquid.

Stir and continue to boil until the liquid thickens. Serve as gravy with the roast.

Chef's Tip: An easy way to peel pearl onions is to slice off the root ends and drop the onions into boiling water for less than a minute. Drain and peel under running cold water.

Serving size: 3 ounces beef with 2 tablespoons gravy, ¼ cup pearl onions	
Each serving	
Glycemic Index	Low
Glycemic Load	2
Calories	239
Fat	14 g
Saturated Fat	5 g
Carbohydrates	6 g
Fiber	0.5 g
Protein	23 g

Tender Baby Back Ribs

Serves 4

¼ cup blackstrap molasses

1 tablespoon paprika

1½ teaspoons chili powder

1½ teaspoons sea salt

¾ teaspoon ground black pepper

¾ teaspoon ground white pepper

¾ teaspoon garlic powder

1 teaspoon ground cumin

½ teaspoon cayenne

½ teaspoon dry mustard

4 pounds baby back ribs*

In a small bowl, mix together the molasses, paprika, chili powder, salt, black pepper, white pepper, garlic powder, cumin, cayenne, and dry mustard. Using your hands, rub the spice mixture all over the ribs. Place in a container large enough to accommodate the rib rack, cover, and marinate in the refrigerator overnight or at least 1 hour. Place the rib rack in the slow cooker. If it does not fit, cut it into sections of two or three bones and stack them, alternating direction between each layer. Cover and cook on low for 7 to 8 hours, or until almost falling off the bone.

Chef's Tip: Four pounds of baby back ribs will feed four very hungry people. If you are trying to keep the caloric value a bit lower, serve two or three ribs per person.

* Ask your butcher to clean the ribs if they haven't already been cleaned. A thick membrane on the bonier side of the ribs becomes tough when cooked, and it doesn't allow for much of the fat from the meat to drip through the meat evenly. If you buy packaged ribs and don't have access to a butcher,

removing the membrane is very simple and there are many online tutorials to guide you.

Serving size: *1 pound per person*	
Each serving	
Glycemic Index	Low
Glycemic Load	8
Calories	786
Fat	38 g
Saturated Fat	13 g
Carbohydrates	18 g
Fiber	1 g
Protein	88 g

Stuffed Cabbage Rolls
Serves 4

1 pound lean ground beef

½ cup uncooked long-grain white rice

1 large egg, beaten

½ cup chopped fresh flat-leaf parsley

3 large cloves garlic, minced

1 teaspoon sea salt

½ teaspoon cracked black pepper

2 tablespoons extra virgin olive oil

1 tablespoon Worcestershire sauce

1 small head green cabbage, core cut out but cabbage head
  left whole

1 large onion, roughly chopped

3 cups low-sodium beef broth (recipe on page 58)

1 (28-ounce) can diced tomatoes

¼ teaspoon red pepper flakes

In a large bowl, combine the ground beef, rice, beaten
egg, parsley, garlic, salt, black pepper, olive oil, and
Worcestershire sauce. Mix well with your hands until the
ingredients are completely combined. Cover and refrigerate
until needed. This part of the dish can be made a day ahead
and the meat will have better flavor.

Bring a large pot of heavily salted water to a boil. Carefully
lower the head of cabbage into the water. As the cabbage
simmers, the leaves will start to loosen after about 3 to 4
minutes and can be pulled off with a pair of tongs. As each
cabbage leaf comes loose, remove it from the simmering
water, and place it in a bowl of cold water. Remove eight
leaves, and reserve the rest of the cabbage for another dish,
such as a soup or a sauté.

When the cabbage leaves are ready, divide the beef and rice mixture into eight small logs. Place the meat at the bottom of the cabbage leaf, where the stem is the thickest, and roll up, loosely folding in the sides as you roll. Line the bottom of your slow cooker with the chopped onion, then top with the cabbage rolls, seam side down. In a large bowl, stir together the beef broth, tomato, and red pepper flakes, and pour on top of the cabbage rolls. Cover and cook on low for 8 to 10 hours or on high for 4 to 6, or until the rice in the meat mixture is cooked.

Serving size: *2 cabbage leaves, 6 ounces meat mixture, 4 tablespoons sauce*	
Each serving	
Glycemic Index	Low
Glycemic Load	6
Calories	506
Fat	33 g
Saturated Fat	11 g
Carbohydrates	22 g
Fiber	3 g
Protein	28 g

Machaca

Serves 8

2 pounds skirt steak, fat trimmed and membrane removed

3 large cloves garlic, minced

½ teaspoon sea salt

½ teaspoon cracked black pepper

½ cup water

2 tablespoons extra virgin olive oil

SALSA

4 cups chopped fresh tomatoes, juices reserved

½ large onion, chopped

½ jalapeño pepper, minced

½ cup packed chopped cilantro

Place the steak along with the garlic, salt, pepper, and water in your slow cooker. Cover and cook on low for 8 to 9 hours or on high for 4 to 4½ hours, or until the meat easily pulls apart. Shred the steak with two forks or by pulling small pieces with your fingers.

To prepare the salsa, mix together the tomato, onion, jalapeño, and cilantro in a large bowl. Next heat a large sauté pan over medium to high heat. Add the oil and then the shredded steak. Brown the meat for 1 to 2 minutes, and then add the fresh salsa. Cover and simmer for about 10 minutes.

Chef's Tip: Machaca is delicious and versatile. Add it to scrambled eggs, use it as a taco or burrito filling, or top a salad with it.

Serving size: ¾ cup	
Each serving	
Glycemic Index	Low
Glycemic Load	1
Calories	269
Fat	14 g
Saturated Fat	5 g
Carbohydrates	4 g
Fiber	1 g
Protein	31 g

Beef Picadillo Lettuce Wraps

Serves 4

1 tablespoon extra virgin olive oil

1 pound lean ground beef

1 cup chopped white onion

2 cups chopped tomatoes

½ cup packed chopped cilantro

1 jalapeño pepper, seeded and finely minced

2 large cloves garlic

1 teaspoon sea salt

1 large head butter lettuce

Heat a large sauté pan over medium to high heat. Once the pan is hot, add the oil and then the ground beef, making sure to break up any large lumps with a spatula. Cook until the meat has browned, about 4 to 5 minutes. Drain the fat from the pan, and add the meat to your slow cooker. Add the onion, tomato, cilantro, jalapeño, garlic, and salt, and mix well. Cover and cook on low for 2 to 3 hours or on high for 1½ to 2 hours. Scoop ¼ cup of the meat mixture into each lettuce leaf, fold it closed and enjoy.

Serving size: 4 ounces beef, 2 lettuce leaves	
Each serving	
Glycemic Index	Low
Glycemic Load	2
Calories	373
Fat	27 g
Saturated Fat	10 g
Carbohydrates	10 g
Fiber	2 g
Protein	22 g

Chapter 8

Vegetarian

Vegetarians, do not fret—we have not forgotten about you! The meatless recipes in this book range from basic slow-cooked vegetables to more gourmet dishes whose flavors will surprise you. A visit to your local farmers market should get you almost all the supplies you will need to make these recipes.

Marinara Sauce

Serves 6

1 (28-ounce) can crushed tomatoes

¼ cup tomato paste

1 cup coarsely chopped yellow onion

2 large cloves garlic, minced

2 bay leaves

⅓ cup chopped fresh basil

¼ cup chopped fresh flat-leaf parsley

1 tablespoon chopped fresh oregano

1 tablespoon finely chopped fresh thyme

1 tablespoon balsamic vinegar

1 teaspoon sea salt

½ teaspoon red pepper flakes

½ teaspoon cracked black pepper

Add all the ingredients to your slow cooker, and stir well. Cover and cook on low for 8 to 9 hours or on high for 4 to 5 hours.

Chef's Tip: Adding the rind from a block of Parmesan cheese to the mixture will give the sauce a delicious and salty touch.

Serving size: *½ cup*	
Each serving	
Glycemic Index	Low
Glycemic Load	1
Calories	52
Fat	0.3 g
Saturated Fat	0.1 g
Carbohydrates	12 g
Fiber	3 g
Protein	3 g

Spaghetti Squash
Serves 6

½ large spaghetti squash (about 1½ pounds)

2 cups water

Cut the ends off the squash. Carefully cut in half lengthwise using a long, sharp knife. Scrape out the seeds and membrane using a metal spoon. Place one half of the squash cut side down in your slow cooker*. Add the water, cover, and cook on low for 6 to 7 hours, or until you can make an indentation in the squash by pressing on the rind with your finger. Remove from the slow cooker and let cool. Using a fork, scrape the flesh into a bowl. Use as a replacement for pasta in your favorite pasta dishes or serve with roasted vegetables topped with cheese shavings.

* Please note that depending on the size of your slow cooker,
  you may or may not be able to fit the entire half of the squash.
  If it does not fit, cut the half into 2 pieces.

Serving size: ½ cup	
Each serving	
Glycemic Index	1
Glycemic Load	21
Calories	0.2 g
Fat	0 g
Saturated Fat	5 g
Carbohydrates	1 g
Fiber	0.5 g
Protein	3 g

Creamed Spinach

Serves 6

3 (10-ounce) packages frozen spinach, thawed and drained
  very well

½ cup chopped white onion

2 large cloves garlic, minced

½ cup low-sodium vegetable broth (recipe on page 56)

½ tablespoon red wine vinegar

¼ teaspoon sea salt

¼ teaspoon cracked black pepper

¼ cup heavy cream

Add the spinach, onion, garlic, broth, vinegar, salt, and
pepper to your slow cooker, and mix well. Cover and cook
on low for 1½ to 2 hours. In the last 30 minutes of cooking
time, stir in the heavy cream and change the setting to high.
Cook uncovered for the final 30 minutes. Before serving,
slightly puree the spinach mixture with an immersion
blender. If you do not have an immersion blender, remove
half the cooked spinach and puree it in an upright blender.
Return the pureed spinach to the slow cooker and stir well.

Serving size: ¾ cup	
Each serving	
Glycemic Index	Low
Glycemic Load	0
Calories	57
Fat	2 g
Saturated Fat	1.2 g
Carbohydrates	8 g
Fiber	4 g
Protein	4 g

Green Enchilada Sauce

Makes 8 cups

1½ pounds green tomatillos, husked and washed

¼ teaspoon cumin seeds

1 cup chopped onion

1 large jalapeño pepper, deseeded if less heat is desired

1 large clove garlic

1 loose bunch cilantro, washed

½ teaspoon sea salt, plus additional, to taste

Quarter the tomatillos and add them to the slow cooker. Heat a large dry skillet over high heat. Add the cumin seeds to the pan and, stirring constantly, toast until fragrant, about 30 seconds. Place the toasted seeds in the slow cooker, and then add the remaining ingredients. Cover and cook on low for 2 to 3 hours or on high for 1 to 1½ hours, or until the onion is soft. Transfer the mixture to a blender, and blend until smooth. Taste and season with additional salt to your liking. If you like your sauce thinner, strain through a fine-mesh strainer if you have one; otherwise any strainer will do.

Serving size: *1 cup*	
Each serving	
Glycemic Index	Very low
Glycemic Load	0
Calories	36
Fat	1 g
Saturated Fat	0.1 g
Carbohydrates	7 g
Fiber	2 g
Protein	1 g

Spinach and Mushroom Enchiladas

Serves 4

8 (6-inch) corn tortillas

1 (10-ounce) package frozen chopped spinach, thawed and
drained very well

2 cups chopped button mushrooms

1 Anaheim chile pepper, seeded and chopped

2 cups shredded Monterey Jack cheese, divided

½ teaspoon ground cumin

½ teaspoon sea salt

½ teaspoon cracked black pepper

4 cups green enchilada sauce (recipe on page 145), divided

¼ cup packed roughly chopped cilantro

Heat a large dry skillet over high heat. Once the pan is hot,
add the tortillas individually and warm each slightly on
both sides. Place the warmed tortillas in a stack inside a
folded kitchen towel to keep warm and set aside.

In a medium bowl, combine the spinach, mushrooms,
Anaheim chile pepper, 1 cup cheese, cumin, salt, and
black pepper. Spread 2 cups green enchilada sauce on the
bottom of the slow cooker. Scoop ½ cup of the vegetable
and cheese mixture into the middle of a warm tortilla. Roll
the tortilla up and place seam side down on top of the
enchilada sauce. Repeat until you have filled all the tortillas.
Top the rolled tortillas with the remaining 2 cups enchilada
sauce and 1 cup cheese. Cover and cook on low for 3 to
3½ hours or on high for 1½ to 2 hours, or until cheese is
melted and enchiladas are heated through. Garnish with the
chopped cilantro.

Serving size: *2 corn tortillas, 1 cup vegetable mixture, ¼ cup enchilada sauce*

Each serving	
Glycemic Index	Low
Glycemic Load	10
Calories	327
Fat	16g
Saturated Fat	9 g
Carbohydrates	33 g
Fiber	6.6 g
Protein	17 g

Vegetarian Green Curry
Serves 6

GREEN CURRY PASTE

1 tablespoon coriander seeds

1 tablespoon cardamom pods

½ tablespoon cumin seeds

1 jalapeño pepper, deseeded if less heat is desired

1 large pitted date

1 inch fresh ginger, peeled

3 cloves garlic

½ cup soy sauce

1 cup packed cilantro

2 stalks lemongrass, outer leaves peeled off, cut into
  ½-inch pieces

VEGETABLE CURRY

2 tablespoons coconut oil

½ cup chopped yellow onion

4 large cloves garlic, minced

1 large red bell pepper, deseeded and cut into 1-inch squares

3 cups Japanese eggplant, halved lengthwise and sliced
  ½ inch thick

2 cups zucchini, sliced ¼ inch thick

3 cups canned coconut milk

2 cups low-sodium vegetable broth (recipe on page 56)

4 tablespoons Thai basil, leaves rolled and thinly sliced,
  for garnish

To toast the coriander, cardamom, and cumin, heat a large
dry sauté pan over high heat. Add the spices to the pan and,
stirring often, toast until fragrant, about 2 to 3 minutes.
Transfer to a blender and add the remaining curry paste
ingredients. Blend until smooth, adding a little water if the
paste is too dry.

To prepare the curry, return the large sauté pan to high heat. Add the coconut oil and then the curry paste. Fry, stirring frequently, until the paste becomes fragrant, about 4 to 5 minutes. Add the onion and garlic, and cook until the onion is translucent, about 2 minutes. Transfer to your slow cooker. Add the bell pepper, eggplant, zucchini, coconut milk, and broth to the slow cooker, and mix well. Cover and cook on low for 5 to 6 hours or on high for 2½ to 3 hours. Garnish each serving with 1 tablespoon Thai basil.

Serving size: 1 cup	
Each serving	
Glycemic Index	Very Low
Glycemic Load	2
Calories	234
Fat	17g
Saturated Fat	16 g
Carbohydrates	17 g
Fiber	4 g
Protein	5 g

Veggie-Stuffed Collard Greens with Tahini Yogurt Sauce

Serves 4

STUFFED COLLARD GREENS

8 large collard green leaves, stems removed

1 large green zucchini, roughly chopped

1 large yellow summer squash, roughly chopped

1 cup packed spinach

1 cup canned cannellini beans, drained and rinsed

1 cup sliced crimini mushrooms

¼ cup chopped red onion

2 large cloves garlic

¼ teaspoon ground white pepper

½ tablespoon Worcestershire sauce

½ cup low-sodium vegetable broth (recipe on page 56)

TAHINI YOGURT SAUCE

1 tablespoon fresh lemon juice

¼ cup tahini

¼ cup 2% Greek yogurt

1 tablespoon chopped fresh flat-leaf parsley

¼ teaspoon sea salt plus additional for blanching greens

¼ teaspoon cracked black pepper

To blanch the collard greens, bring a large pot of heavily salted water to a boil. Dip the leaves into the boiling water for about 30 seconds and then immediately plunge them into a bowl of ice water. Repeat until all the leaves are blanched.

In a food processor, combine the zucchini, squash, spinach, beans, mushrooms, red onion, garlic, white pepper, and Worcestershire sauce, and pulse until the vegetables are very small and start to puree. Scrape out into a bowl and set aside. Spread out the blanched collard greens leaves and place ½ cup of the vegetable mixture in the shape of a log close on the bottom center edge of each leaf. Fold the sides over, then roll up tightly, tucking in the sides as you go. Place seam side down in the slow cooker, fitting the stuffed leaves in snug layers. Add the broth, cover, and cook on low for 3½ to 4 hours or on high for 2 to 2½ hours.

Meanwhile, whisk together the tahini yogurt sauce ingredients, and drizzle the sauce over the cooked rolls when serving.

Serving size: *2 stuffed collard green leaves*	
Each serving	
Glycemic Index	Low
Glycemic Load	4
Calories	135
Fat	0.6 g
Saturated Fat	0.1 g
Carbohydrates	25 g
Fiber	7 g
Protein	10 g

Curried Red Lentils

Serves 8

½ teaspoon ground cumin

2 cups red lentils

1 (16-ounce) can diced tomatoes

7 cups low-sodium vegetable broth (recipe on page 56)

1 cup canned coconut milk

1 large carrot, finely chopped

½ large white onion, finely chopped

2 celery stalks, finely chopped

1 inch fresh ginger, peeled and finely chopped

1 tablespoon tomato paste

1 tablespoon fresh lemon juice

2 bay leaves

¼ teaspoon red pepper flakes

1 tablespoon curry powder

1 teaspoon turmeric

1 teaspoon sea salt

Toast the cumin: Heat a small sauté pan over medium heat, and add the cumin when the pan is hot. Stir constantly until fragrant, about 1 minute. Remove from the heat and place in the slow cooker. Add all the remaining ingredients to the slow cooker, and mix well. Cover and cook on low for 8 to 10 hours or on high for 5 to 6 hours or until lentils have absorbed all the liquid and are soft and falling apart.

Serving size: *1 cup*	
Each serving	
Glycemic Index	Low
Glycemic Load	6
Calories	271
Fat	6 g
Saturated Fat	4 g
Carbohydrates	40 g
Fiber	9 g
Protein	15 g

Garlicky Brussels Sprouts

Serves 4

1 pound brussels sprouts, trimmed and halved

2 large cloves garlic, minced

2 tablespoons extra virgin olive oil

½ teaspoon sea salt

½ teaspoon cracked black pepper

In a large bowl, toss the brussels sprouts with the garlic, olive oil, salt, and pepper. Transfer to the slow cooker, cover, and cook on low for 4 to 5 hours or on high for 2 to 2½ hours, or until the consistency of the brussels sprouts is to your liking. Cooking them on high for 2½ hours will leave them very soft.

Serving size: ½ cup	
Each serving	
Glycemic Index	Low
Glycemic Load	0
Calories	81
Fat	7 g
Saturated Fat	1 g
Carbohydrates	4 g
Fiber	2 g
Protein	2 g

Cheesy Broccoli Gratin

Serves 6

6 cups broccoli florets

¼ teaspoon dry mustard

⅛ teaspoon ground white pepper

½ teaspoon sea salt

1 cup low-sodium vegetable broth (recipe on page 56)

1 tablespoon unsalted butter

½ cup gluten-free bread crumbs

½ teaspoon chopped fresh thyme

1 teaspoon chopped fresh flat-leaf parsley

2 tablespoons amaranth flour*

½ cup heavy cream

1 cup shredded sharp cheddar cheese

In a large bowl, toss the broccoli with the dry mustard, white pepper, and salt. Spread the seasoned broccoli evenly in the bottom of your slow cooker, and add the broth. Cover and cook on low for 5 to 6 hours or on high for 2½ to 3 hours.

While the broccoli cooks, heat a medium sauté pan over high heat. Melt the butter, and then add the bread crumbs, thyme, and parsley. Stir often until the bread crumbs turn golden brown and are fragrant, about 3 to 4 minutes. Remove from the pan and set aside.

In a small bowl, whisk the flour and heavy cream. In the last 30 minutes of cooking time for the broccoli, remove the slow cooker cover, drizzle the cream and flour mixture over top, and then sprinkle on the cheese and finally the toasted bread crumbs. Cook uncovered on high for 20 to 30 minutes, or until the cheese melts and the sauce thickens.

* Amaranth flour can be found at most health food stores. It is a gluten-free flour made from amaranth seeds and can be used in place of all-purpose flour to thicken sauces. If you cannot find amaranth flour, you can substitute it with brown rice flour or garbanzo bean flour.

Serving size: 1 cup	
Each serving	
Glycemic Index	Low
Glycemic Load	4
Calories	233
Fat	16 g
Saturated Fat	10 g
Carbohydrates	14 g
Fiber	3 g
Protein	9 g

Saag Paneer with Garbanzo Beans

Serves 4

12 ounces fresh paneer cheese,* cut into 1-inch cubes

1 tablespoon vegetable oil

½ teaspoon cayenne

½ teaspoon turmeric

½ teaspoon sea salt

1 (16-ounce) package frozen chopped spinach, thawed and
  drained very well

½ large yellow onion, diced

2 large cloves garlic, minced

1 inch fresh ginger, peeled and grated

1 (15-ounce) can garbanzo beans, drained and rinsed

1 teaspoon ground cumin

1 teaspoon curry powder

1 tablespoon ground coriander

½ teaspoon garam masala*

½ cup water

In a small bowl, combine the paneer cheese, vegetable oil,
cayenne, turmeric, and salt. Set aside to marinate while
preparing the remaining ingredients. Heat a large nonstick
sauté pan over medium heat. Once the pan is hot, add
the marinated paneer, and cook until brown, about 3 to 4
minutes on each side. (If you don't have a large pan, cook
in batches, as overcrowding will keep the paneer from
browning.) Remove and drain on paper towels.

Place the spinach in your slow cooker. Add the onion,
garlic, ginger, garbanzo beans, cumin, curry powder,
coriander, garam masala, and water, and stir well. Place the
browned paneer cheese on top, cover, and cook on low for
about 4 to 5 hours or on high for 1½ to 2 hours.

* Paneer cheese and garam masala can be found in most Middle Eastern markets and sometimes in the international aisle of your grocery store.

Serving size: *1 cup*	
Each serving	
Glycemic Index	Low
Glycemic Load	18
Calories	365
Fat	8 g
Saturated Fat	1.5 g
Carbohydrates	58 g
Fiber	11 g
Protein	19 g

Quinoa-Stuffed Zucchini

Serves 4

4 large zucchini

1 cup cooked quinoa*

⅛ cup chopped red onion

¼ cup chopped jarred roasted red peppers

⅛ cup crumbled feta cheese

1 tablespoon red wine vinegar

2 tablespoons extra virgin olive oil, divided

½ teaspoon sea salt

cracked black pepper, to taste

2 tablespoons chopped fresh flat-leaf parsley

¼ teaspoon dried Italian herbs, such as thyme, basil, and
   rosemary

Using a paring knife, cut the top ¼ inch off each zucchini, lengthwise. Insert the tip of a teaspoon or melon baller near the end of the zucchini, push down, and begin to remove the center. Continue scooping until most of the center is removed.

To prepare the quinoa salad, thoroughly combine the cooked quinoa, red onion, roasted red pepper, feta cheese, vinegar, 1 tablespoon olive oil, dried Italian herbs, salt, and pepper in a medium bowl. Scoop ¼ cup of the quinoa salad into each hollowed-out zucchini, and carefully place each stuffed zucchini in the bottom of the slow cooker. Drizzle the remaining 1 tablespoon olive oil over the top of each zucchini. Cover and cook on low for 3 to 4 hours or on high for 1½ to 2 hours, or until the zucchini is easily pierced with a fork. Serve warm and sprinkle with parsley.

* To cook the quinoa, rinse it first in a fine-mesh strainer if it is
   not pre-rinsed. In a small pot over high heat, combine 1 part

quinoa to 2 parts water with a dash of sea salt. Once the pot comes to a boil, reduce the heat to low and cover. Simmer for 12 to 15 minutes or until the grains start to uncoil, at which point they absorb all the water and become fluffy. Remove from the heat, let stand with lid on for 5 minutes, and then fluff with a fork. Note that 1 cup uncooked quinoa plus 2 cups water yield about 3 cups cooked quinoa.

Serving size: *1 large zucchini, 1/4 cup quinoa salad*	
Each serving	
Glycemic Index	Low
Glycemic Load	7
Calories	183
Fat	10 g
Saturated Fat	2 g
Carbohydrates	22 g
Fiber	3 g
Protein	5 g

Buckwheat and Pesto–Stuffed Portobello Mushrooms

Serves 4

4 large portobello mushrooms, about 4 inches in diameter,
  stems removed

¼ cup balsamic vinegar

1 teaspoon sea salt, divided

1 teaspoon cracked black pepper, divided

1 cup packed basil leaves

4 tablespoons shredded Parmesan cheese

½ cup toasted pine nuts

2 large cloves garlic

⅛ cup extra virgin olive oil

1 cup cooked buckwheat*

Remove the stems from the mushrooms and, using a
teaspoon in a circular motion, scoop out the gills. Wipe
the mushroom caps with a damp towel to remove any dirt.
Place the mushrooms, cap-side facing down in a shallow
baking dish. Evenly drizzle the balsamic vinegar over the
insides of the mushrooms, season with ½ teaspoon salt and
½ teaspoon pepper, and set aside. Prepare the pesto by
adding the basil, Parmesan, pine nuts, garlic, olive oil, and
the remaining salt and pepper to a small food processor
or blender, and pulsing until the mixture becomes a
thick paste. Place the cooked buckwheat in a small bowl,
and pour the pesto over top. Mix well and evenly scoop
buckwheat mixture into each mushroom cap until full.

Spray the inside of the slow cooker with nonstick spray.
Place the mushrooms caps inside the slow cooker. Cover
and cook on low for 4 to 5 hours or on high for 2 to 2½

hours or until mushrooms are soft and can be easily pierced with a fork.

* To cook buckwheat, use 1 part buckwheat to 2 parts liquid. Place the buckwheat in a pot with water, cover, and bring to a boil. Reduce the heat to low, and simmer until tender, about 15 to 20 minutes. Remove from the heat, let stand with the lid on for 5 minutes, then fluff with a fork. Kasha, or toasted buckwheat, requires significantly less cooking time than untoasted buckwheat, so be sure to read the label when purchasing. Note that 1 cup uncooked buckwheat plus 2 cups water yield about 4 cups cooked buckwheat.

Serving size: *1 mushroom cap, ¼ cup buckwheat and pesto stuffing*	
Each serving	
Glycemic Index	Low
Glycemic Load	14
Calories	428
Fat	28
Saturated Fat	4 g
Carbohydrates	38 g
Fiber	6 g
Protein	12 g

Italian-Style Stuffed Tomatoes

Serves 4

1 cup cooked quinoa*

1 cup packed roughly chopped fresh spinach

¼ cup roughly chopped toasted walnuts

1 tablespoon roughly chopped capers

1 tablespoon chopped fresh flat-leaf parsley

1 teaspoon chopped fresh oregano or ¼ teaspoon dried
  oregano

1 teaspoon sea salt

½ teaspoon cracked black pepper

4 large tomatoes, tops cut off and pulp scooped out with spoon

½ cup shredded part-skim mozzarella cheese

4 tablespoons gluten-free bread crumbs

2 tablespoons extra virgin olive oil

In a small bowl, combine the cooked quinoa, spinach,
walnuts, capers, parsley, and oregano. Season with the
salt and pepper. Scoop one quarter of this quinoa mixture
into each tomato half, patting it down if necessary. Place
the stuffed tomato halves in your slow cooker. Sprinkle 2
tablespoons mozzarella cheese and then 1 tablespoon bread
crumbs on top of each tomato. Finally drizzle ½ teaspoon
olive oil over each tomato. Cover and cook on low for 3½ to
4 hours or on high for 1½ to 2 hours, or until the tomatoes
are tender but still holding their shape.

* Rinse the quinoa in a fine-mesh strainer if it is not pre-rinsed.
  In a small pot over high heat, combine 1 part quinoa to 2
  parts water with a dash of sea salt. Once the pot comes to a
  boil, reduce the heat to low and cover. Simmer for 12 to 15
  minutes or until the grains start to uncoil, at which point they
  absorb all the water and become fluffy. Remove from the heat,
  let stand with lid on for 5 minutes, and then fluff with a fork.

Note that 1 cup uncooked quinoa plus 2 cups water yield about 3 cups cooked quinoa.

Serving size: *1 tomato, ¼ cup quinoa and veggie mixture*	
Each serving	
Glycemic Index	Low
Glycemic Load	9
Calories	230
Fat	9 g
Saturated Fat	1.8 g
Carbohydrates	30 g
Fiber	5 g
Protein	11 g

Vegetarian Lasagna
Serves 8

1 medium eggplant, sliced into ¼-inch rounds

1 pound portobello mushrooms, stems and gills removed, sliced ¼ inch thick

8 ounces zucchini, sliced lengthwise ¼ inch thick

2 tablespoons extra virgin olive oil

½ teaspoon minced garlic

1½ teaspoons sea salt

1 teaspoon cracked black pepper

2 cups low-fat ricotta cheese

2 tablespoons nonfat milk

¼ cup freshly grated Parmesan cheese, plus 1 tablespoon for garnish

¼ cup plus 1 tablespoon fresh basil, sliced into thin ribbons

2 tablespoons chopped fresh flat-leaf parsley, divided

1 large egg, beaten

3 cups low-sodium marinara sauce (recipe on page 142), divided

9 whole wheat lasagna noodles, uncooked

4 cups packed, roughly chopped fresh spinach

2 cups grated part-skim mozzarella cheese

Preheat the oven to 375°F. Spray two baking sheets with nonstick cooking spray, and arrange the eggplant, mushroom, and zucchini slices in a single layer on the sheets. Brush olive oil on the vegetables, and sprinkle with the garlic, salt, and pepper. Bake for 8 to 10 minutes, or until vegetables have browned.

To cut the basil, stack a few leaves, roll them tightly into a tight tube, and slice them very thinly. While the vegetables are roasting, mix together the ricotta cheese, milk, ¼ cup

Parmesan cheese, ¼ cup basil, 1 tablespoon parsley, and beaten egg in a large bowl.

Spread ¼ cup marinara sauce in the bottom of the slow cooker. Layer the ingredients on top of the marinara base as follows: three lasagna noodles, half of the ricotta cheese mixture, a layer of baked vegetables, a layer of spinach, one third of the remaining marinara sauce, and one third of the mozzarella cheese. Repeat the layers. Top with the remaining three lasagna noodles and the remaining marinara sauce. Cover and cook on low for 5 to 6 hours or on high for 2½ to 3 hours. In the last 20 minutes of cooking, uncover and sprinkle on the remaining mozzarella cheese. Garnish with the remaining 1 tablespoon parsley and the remaining 1 tablespoon basil.

Serving size: 8 ounces	
Each serving	
Glycemic Index	Low
Glycemic Load	13
Calories	458
Fat	22 g
Saturated Fat	11 g
Carbohydrates	37 g
Fiber	5 g
Protein	30 g

Chapter 9

Desserts

There is nothing better than fresh, delicious fruit for dessert. But what about the times you're craving something sweet and gooey, or sweet and comforting, or something simple that hits your sweet spot? Creating slow cooker dessert recipes with little to no sugar is a challenge. After doing extensive research, we learned that coconut palm sugar is a great low-GI option. It is all natural and, although a tad high on the caloric scale, will not cause a spike in blood sugar as other forms of sugar will. You can find coconut palm sugar at your local health food store or online.

Almond and Carob Chip Bake

Serves 8

1 cup unsalted, smooth almond butter

¼ cup coconut palm sugar

1 teaspoon baking soda

½ teaspoon almond extract

2 egg whites, beaten

4 tablespoons carob chips

¼ teaspoon Himalayan pink salt or sea salt

In a medium bowl, combine the almond butter, coconut palm sugar, baking soda, almond extract, and egg whites. Once the ingredients are incorporated, stir in the carob chips. Spray the inside of the slow cooker with nonstick spray. Press the mixture into the slow cooker into an even layer and sprinkle the salt over top. Cover and cook on low for 2½ to 3 hours, or until inserted knife comes out clean. Serve warm or cooled.

Serving size: *1 2-inch square*	
Each serving	
Glycemic Index	Low
Glycemic Load	2
Calories	237
Fat	18 g
Saturated Fat	2 g
Carbohydrates	14 g
Fiber	4 g
Protein	10 g

Fresh Apple Compote
Serves 4

5 cups chopped unpeeled Fuji or Cameo apples

1 tablespoon ground cinnamon

½ teaspoon ground ginger

⅛ teaspoon ground cloves

2 tablespoons fresh lemon juice

Add all the ingredients to the slow cooker, and mix well.
Cover and cook on low for 4 to 5 hours or on high for 2 to
2½ hours, or until the apples have broken down and are
soft. At the end of the cooking time, or when the apples
have reached a consistency you like, mash them with a fork
or potato masher. Serve warm or cold.

Chef's Tip: Leaving the skin on the apples provides more
texture as well as more fiber, which slows down digestion,
causing slower conversion of carbohydrates to glucose and
therefore less of a spike in blood sugar.

Serving size: ¼ cup	
Each serving	
Glycemic Index	Low
Glycemic Load	8
Calories	94
Fat	0.2 g
Saturated Fat	0.1 g
Carbohydrates	25 g
Fiber	4 g
Protein	0.3 g

Peanut Butter Banana Chocolate Chip Bars

Serves 8

2 cups gluten-free old-fashioned oats

⅔ cup almond meal

⅓ cup plus 2 tablespoons shredded unsweetened coconut, divided

½ cup 70% or darker chocolate chips

½ teaspoon sea salt

3 small ripe bananas, mashed (about 3 cups)

½ teaspoon vanilla extract

¼ cup chunky or creamy unsalted peanut butter

¼ cup unsweetened applesauce

¾ teaspoon ground cinnamon, divided

In a medium bowl, combine the oats, almond meal, ⅓ cup shredded coconut, chocolate chips, and salt. In another large bowl, combine the bananas, vanilla, peanut butter, applesauce, and ½ teaspoon cinnamon, and mash thoroughly using a potato masher or fork. Add the oat mixture to the banana mixture, and mix well.

Spray the inside of the slow cooker with nonstick spray, and pour the batter into the slow cooker. Top with the remaining 2 tablespoons coconut and ¼ teaspoon cinnamon. Place a large paper towel on top of the slow cooker and then place the lid over the paper towel. Cook on low for 2 hours or on high for 1 hour. Let cool completely before slicing into bars.

Serving size: *1 2-inch square*	
Each serving	
Glycemic Index	Low
Glycemic Load	14
Calories	314
Fat	17 g
Saturated Fat	6 g
Carbohydrates	38 g
Fiber	6 g
Protein	7 g

Dairy-Free Chocolate Peanut Butter Custard

Serves 4

1½ cups coconut milk

2 large eggs

¼ cup unsweetened dark cocoa powder

¼ teaspoon vanilla extract

⅛ teaspoon sea salt

¼ teaspoon ground cinnamon

4 teaspoon unsalted smooth peanut butter

2 tablespoon pure honey

Spray four 7-ounce ramekins with nonstick spray. Heat the coconut milk in a small pot over medium heat. While the milk heats, start whisking the eggs in a medium bowl, then add the cocoa powder, vanilla, salt, and cinnamon, and continue whisking the mixture until smooth. Once the milk is steaming and about to boil, remove it from the heat. Slowly drizzle in about ⅛ cup hot milk into the egg mixture, and whisk that in. Pour in the remaining milk while whisking, and continue whisking until there are no lumps. Pour mixture into greased ramekins until about ¼-inch below the top.

Arrange the ramekins in the slow cooker, being cautious not to spill any of the custard. Carefully pour in just enough hot water to reach halfway up the sides of the ramekins. Cover and cook on high for 45 to 55 minutes, or until the custard has set and jiggles slightly in the center. Turn off the slow cooker and let the ramekins sit for 5 minutes. Uncover the slow cooker, remove the ramekins, and let the custard cool at room temperature. Enjoy once cooled or refrigerate overnight.

While the custard cooks, thoroughly combine the peanut butter and honey in a small bowl. Spread 1 teaspoon of this mixture on top of each cooled custard. Sprinkle with a dash of cinnamon or serve with a couple of banana slices.*

* Keep in mind that adding banana slices will slightly change the nutrition facts for this recipe.

Serving size: 6 ounces	
Each serving	
Glycemic Index	Low
Glycemic Load	4
Calories	132
Fat	8 g
Saturated Fat	4 g
Carbohydrates	13 g
Fiber	2 g
Protein	4 g

Gluten-Free Apple Raisin Crumble
Serves 8

APPLE RAISIN MIXTURE

1 pound Granny Smith apples, peeled and chopped into
  ½-inch pieces

2 teaspoons melted unsalted butter

1 tablespoon fresh lemon juice

½ cup golden raisins

1 teaspoon ground cinnamon

½ teaspoon ground ginger

⅛ teaspoon ground nutmeg

CRUMBLE TOPPING

½ cup oat flour

⅓ cup almond meal

¼ cup chopped walnuts

3 tablespoons unsalted butter, very cold and cut into quarters

½ teaspoon ground cinnamon

Place the chopped apples in a medium bowl. Add the
melted butter, lemon juice, raisins, cinnamon, ginger, and
nutmeg, and toss until the apple is evenly coated. Arrange
in an even layer in the bottom of your slow cooker.

To make the crumble, combine the oat flour, almond meal,
and walnuts in a medium bowl. Using a fork or your fingers,
cut the butter into the crumble mixture until there are small
lumps. Evenly spread the crumble topping over the apple
layer, cover, and cook on low for 3 to 4 hours or on high
for 1½ to 2½ hours. Turn the slow cooker off, uncover, and
allow the crust to harden and dry a bit, about 20 minutes.

Serving size: ¾ cup	
Each serving	
Glycemic Index	Low to Medium
Glycemic Load	7
Calories	154
Fat	11 g
Saturated Fat	5 g
Carbohydrates	15 g
Fiber	2 g
Protein	2 g

Stuffed Green Apples

Serves 4

4 medium Granny Smith apples, unpeeled and cored with
  bottom still in place

3 tablespoons fresh lemon juice

½ cup unsalted smooth almond butter

½ cup finely chopped dried apricots, divided

2 tablespoons ground cinnamon, plus more for topping

⅛ teaspoon ground nutmeg

⅛ teaspoon sea salt

4 teaspoons unsweetened shredded coconut

Brush the inside of each cored apple with lemon juice. In a
small bowl, mix together the almond butter, 4 tablespoons
chopped apricot, cinnamon, nutmeg, and salt. Spoon the
almond butter mixture into the apples. Top each apple with
1 tablespoon chopped apricots, a sprinkling of cinnamon,
and 1 teaspoon shredded coconut. Place the cored apples
in your slow cooker, and pour water in the bottom. Cover
and cook on low for 2 to 3 hours, or on high for 1 to 1½
hours, or until the apples are soft when pierced with a fork.

Chef's Tip: To core an apple, cut in a wide, circular motion
all the way around the top of the apple toward the base. Pop
the top off, and cut or scoop away remaining seeds and any
tough pieces connected to the core using a teaspoon.

Serving size: *1 apple, 4 tablespoons almond butter and apricot mixture, 1 teaspoon coconut*

Each serving	
Glycemic Index	Low
Glycemic Load	8
Calories	334
Fat	20 g
Saturated Fat	2 g
Carbohydrates	43 g
Fiber	11 g
Protein	6 g

Gluten-Free Mexican Chocolate Torte

Serves 6

¼ cup gluten-free oat flour

6 tablespoons unsweetened dark cocoa powder

⅛ teaspoon ground cinnamon

⅛ teaspoon cayenne

⅛ teaspoon sea salt

4 large eggs

½ cup coconut palm sugar

8 ounces unsweetened plain applesauce

½ cup plain whole-milk yogurt

1 teaspoon vanilla extract

1 tablespoon orange zest

2 tablespoons carob chips

Combine the oat flour, cocoa powder, cinnamon, cayenne, and salt, and set aside. With an electric mixer on medium-high speed, beat the eggs until foamy and thick. Gradually add the palm sugar until the mixture is frothy and pale. Whisk in the applesauce, yogurt, vanilla, and orange zest. Add the flour mixture to the egg mixture, and whisk until the dry ingredients are incorporated.

Spray the inside of your slow cooker with nonstick spray. Pour the batter into the slow cooker and sprinkle carob chips evenly over the top. Lay two paper towels over the top of the cooker to absorb condensation, then place the lid on top of the paper towels. Cook on low for 50 minutes, or until an inserted knife comes out clean.

Serving Suggestion: Serve warm with fresh strawberries or raspberries.*

* Please note that adding strawberries or raspberries will slightly change the nutrition facts for this recipe.

Serving size: *4 ounces*	
Each serving	
Glycemic Index	Low
Glycemic Load	9
Calories	189
Fat	7 g
Saturated Fat	3 g
Carbohydrates	30 g
Fiber	3 g
Protein	7 g

Berry Cobbler
Serves 6

BERRY MIXTURE

1 (16-ounce) package frozen berry medley

2 tablespoons cornstarch

2 tablespoons coconut palm sugar

¼ cup water

¼ teaspoon vanilla extract

1 tablespoon lemon zest

CRUMBLE TOPPING

½ cup gluten-free oat flour

⅛ cup uncooked quinoa

½ tablespoon flax seeds

¼ teaspoon ground nutmeg

⅛ cup walnut pieces

¼ teaspoon ground cinnamon

5 tablespoons cold unsalted butter, quartered

Add the frozen berries, cornstarch, sugar, water, vanilla, and lemon zest to your slow cooker, and stir well. To make the crumble, combine the oat flour, uncooked quinoa, flax seeds, nutmeg, walnuts, and cinnamon in a small bowl. Using a fork or your fingers, cut the butter into the flour mixture until there are small lumps. Evenly spread the crumble topping over the berry mixture. Cover and cook on low for 4 to 4½ hours or on high for 2 to 2½ hours. Remove the lid after the allotted time to allow for the crust to harden and dry a bit.

Serving size: ½ cup	
Each serving	
Glycemic Index	Low
Glycemic Load	14
Calories	273
Fat	14 g
Saturated Fat	6 g
Carbohydrates	36 g
Fiber	4 g
Protein	4 g

Pumpkin Custard

Serves 4

1 (15-ounce) can pumpkin puree

1½ cups half and half

2 large eggs

¼ cup coconut palm sugar

1 tablespoon ground cinnamon

½ teaspoon ground nutmeg

¼ teaspoon ground cloves

¼ teaspoon ground ginger

1 teaspoon vanilla extract

Add all the ingredients to a blender, and blend until smooth. Lightly grease four 7-ounce ramekins with nonstick spray, and pour an equal amount of batter into each ramekin, about ¼-inch below the top. Arrange the ramekins in the slow cooker, being cautious not to spill any of the custard. Carefully pour in just enough hot water to reach halfway up the sides of the ramekins. Cover and cook on high for 2 to 2½ hours, or until the custard has set and jiggles slightly in the center. Turn off the slow cooker and let the ramekins sit for 5 minutes. Uncover the slow cooker, remove the ramekins, and let the custard cool at room temperature. Enjoy once slightly cooled or place in refrigerator overnight.

Serving size: *6 ounces*	
Each serving	
Glycemic Index	Low
Glycemic Load	7
Calories	216
Fat	15 g
Saturated Fat	8 g
Carbohydrates	19 g
Fiber	4 g
Protein	7 g

Pear and Ginger Compote

Serves 4

2 pounds very ripe Bosc or Bartlett pears, peeled and cut into
  ½-inch pieces

½ inch fresh ginger, peeled and finely chopped

1 tablespoon ground cinnamon

½ cup water

1 tablespoon fresh lemon juice

Add all the ingredients to your slow cooker, and mix well.
Cover and cook on low for 3½ to 4 hours, or until fruit
pieces have broken down. If you prefer a less chunky
compote, use a potato masher to mash the cooked pears.

Serving size: *½ cup*	
Each serving	
Glycemic Index	Low
Glycemic Load	7
Calories	107
Fat	0.3 g
Saturated Fat	0 g
Carbohydrates	28 g
Fiber	6 g
Protein	1 g

Ricotta Cakes with Fresh Figs

Serves 4

2 large egg whites plus 1 large egg yolk

⅛ teaspoon cream of tartar

½ teaspoon vanilla extract

1 cup ricotta cheese

1 tablespoon pure maple syrup

1 teaspoon ground cinnamon

¼ teaspoon ground cloves

4 large figs, stems removed and thinly sliced

4 teaspoons roughly chopped toasted pistachios

In a small bowl, use an electric mixer to beat the egg whites, cream of tartar, and vanilla extract until the egg whites are fluffy and form soft peaks. In a separate medium bowl, mix together the ricotta, egg yolk, maple syrup, cinnamon, and cloves, and mash with a fork to break up any lumps. Using a spatula, fold the egg whites into the ricotta mixture in batches until you have incorporated all of them.

Grease four 7-ounce ramekins with nonstick spray, and evenly scoop the ricotta batter into each one, making sure to level off the tops. Arrange the ramekins in the slow cooker, place two paper towels over the slow cooker, then place the lid on top of the paper towels. Cook on low for 7 to 8 hours or on high for 3½ to 4 hours, or until a toothpick inserted into the cake comes out clean. Serve each cake with slices of fig and a sprinkling of pistachios on top.

Serving size: *7 ounces cake, 1 fig*	
Each serving	
Glycemic Index	Low
Glycemic Load	6
Calories	186
Fat	9 g
Saturated Fat	4 g
Carbohydrates	18 g
Fiber	3 g
Protein	12 g

Upside Down Pear Chocolate Cake

Serves 6

4 large Bosc pears, peeled, very thinly sliced

¼ cup gluten-free oat flour

6 tablespoons unsweetened dark cocoa powder

⅛ teaspoon ground cinnamon

⅛ teaspoon salt

4 small eggs

1 cup unsweetened applesauce

½ cup plain whole-milk yogurt

1 teaspoon vanilla extract

2 tablespoons carob chips

Spray the inside of your slow cooker with nonstick spray.
Lay the pear slices in the bottom of the slow cooker,
shingling them in neat rows.

In a small bowl, mix together the oat flour, cocoa powder,
cinnamon, and salt. Crack the eggs into a medium bowl
and, using an electric mixer, beat until foamy and thick.
Gradually add the applesauce, yogurt, and vanilla. Add
the flour mixture to the egg mixture in small batches,
continuing to beat with mixer until the dry ingredients are
incorporated.

Pour the batter in an even layer on top of the pear slices and
sprinkle evenly with the carob chips. Lay two paper towels
over the slow cooker then place the lid on top. Cook on low
for 50 minutes, or until an inserted knife comes out clean.
Carefully scoop out the cake with a large, flat spatula to
preserve the rows of pears. Invert the slices onto plates so
the pears are on top.

Serving size: *4 ounces*	
Each serving	
Glycemic Index	Low
Glycemic Load	7
Calories	139
Fat	4 g
Saturated Fat	2 g
Carbohydrates	23 g
Fiber	5 g
Protein	6 g

Vanilla Espresso Custard

Serves 4

4 large eggs

2 cups whole milk

⅛ cup coconut palm sugar

1 teaspoon vanilla extract

Seeds from ½ vanilla bean, halved bean reserved

1 teaspoon instant espresso powder

¼ teaspoon salt

In a medium bowl, whisk the eggs well. In a medium pot, whisk together the milk, sugar, vanilla extract, vanilla bean seeds, halved vanilla bean, espresso powder, and salt. Cook over medium heat, stirring frequently to avoid scorching, until the milk approaches a simmer. Remove from the heat. Whisk the eggs continuously while drizzling in 2 tablespoons of the hot milk, and continue whisking until the mixture is frothy. Remove the vanilla bean from the milk and slowly drizzle in the remaining hot milk in a steady stream while continuing to whisk, to avoid cooking the eggs.

Lightly grease four 7-ounce ramekins with nonstick spray. Pour the custard into the ramekins until ¼-inch below the top, and carefully transfer to the slow cooker. Add just enough hot water to reach halfway up the sides of the ramekins. Cover and cook on high for 45 to 55 minutes, or until the custard has set and jiggles slightly in the center. Turn off the slow cooker and let the ramekins sit for 5 minutes. Uncover the slow cover, remove the ramekins, and let the custard cool at room temperature. Enjoy once cooled or refrigerate overnight.

Serving size: 6 ounces	
Each serving	
Glycemic Index	Low
Glycemic Load	6
Calories	184
Fat	9 g
Saturated Fat	4 g
Carbohydrates	18 g
Fiber	0 g
Protein	10 g

Strawberry and Basil Compote

Serves 4

1 pound strawberries, hulled and quartered

⅓ cup basil, cut into thin ribbons

2 tablespoons fresh lemon juice

1 tablespoon balsamic vinegar

Add the strawberries to your slow cooker. To cut the basil, stack a few leaves, roll them tightly into a tight tube, and slice them very thinly. Add the basil, lemon juice, and balsamic vinegar to the slow cooker, and mix well. Cover and cook on low for 3 to 4 hours, or until the strawberries have broken down. If you prefer a less chunky compote, use a potato masher to mash the cooked strawberries.

Serving Suggestion: This compote is delicious and very versatile. Serve it on top of your favorite yogurt for breakfast or, for a fresh twist, on top of grilled chicken breasts.

Serving size: ½ cup	
Each serving	
Glycemic Index	Low
Glycemic Load	2
Calories	41
Fat	0.5 g
Saturated Fat	0 g
Carbohydrates	9 g
Fiber	3 g
Protein	1 g

Appendix

Appendix A

Glycemic Index

Here is a chart listing the glycemic index number for the ingredients used in our recipes along with some other common foods. This can help you keep in mind what foods are good to eat every day and what common foods you might want to eat only on occasion.

Vegetables	Glycemic Index
Acorn squash	75
Artichoke hearts	15
Arugula	5
Avocado	0
Bell pepper	40
Bok choy	10
Broccoli	10
Brussels sprouts	25
Butter lettuce	15
Butternut squash	51
Cabbage	<10
Carrot	39
Cassava	94
Chard	5
Chipotle chile pepper	5
Collard greens	5
Eggplant	10
English peas	22
Fava beans	63

Vegetables Continued	Glycemic Index
Garlic	<5
Green olives	15
Green onion	<10
Green peas	54
Herbs, fresh and dried	<5
Leek	10
Mushrooms, Chanterelle	10
Mushrooms, Crimini	10
Mushrooms, Portobello	10
Onion	10
Parsnip	52
Pasilla chile pepper	40
Potato, new	80
Potato, red	89
Potato, white	69
Pumpkin	64
Radish	<10
Romaine lettuce	5
Shallot	10
Spinach	15
Squash, spaghetti	20
Squash, yellow	25
Sweet corn	60
Sweet potato	44
Taro	48
Tomatillo	38
Tomato	38
Tomato paste	10
Yam	37
Zucchini	50

Fruits	Glycemic Index
Apple	35
Applesauce	53
Apricot, dried	32
Apricot, fresh	34
Banana	51
Blackberries	32
Blueberries	53
Breadfruit	68
Cantaloupe	65
Chayote fruit	31
Cherries	63
Dates	42
Fig	35
Frozen berries	38
Grapefruit, ruby red	47
Grapes, black	59
Kiwi	58
Lemon juice	<5
Lime juice	<5
Mandarin orange	47
Mango	51
Nectarine	43
Orange	43
Peach	42
Pear	36
Pineapple	59
Plantain	55
Raisins	64
Raspberries	35
Strawberries	40
Watermelon	76

Grains	Glycemic Index
Arborio rice	69
Barley	25
Bread crumbs, gluten-free	45
Brown rice	48
Buckwheat	54
Flour, all-purpose	44
Flour, oat	58
Oats, steel cut	58
Polenta	69
Red rice	59
Sprouted grain bread, Ezekiel	45
Tortilla, corn	52
Tortilla, whole wheat	30
White rice, basmati	44
White rice, jasmine	89
White rice, long grain	50
White rice, medium grain	78
Whole wheat pasta	55
Wild rice	45

Nuts, Seeds, Beans, and Legumes	Glycemic Index
Almond meal	0
Almond milk	0
Almonds	0
Beans, black	20
Beans, black-eyed	33
Beans, butter	36
Beans, cannellini	31
Beans, garbanzo	28
Beans, mung	31
Beans, navy	31
Beans, pinto	33
Beans, red kidney	27
Beans, white kidney	14
Cashew nuts	22
Flax seed	32

Nuts, Seeds, Beans, and Legumes *Continued*	Glycemic Index
Hominy	40
Lentils, brown	29
Lentils, green	37
Lentils, red	21
Marrowfat peas	47
Mixed nuts	24
Peanut butter	14
Peanuts	7
Pigeon peas	22
Pine nuts	15
Pistachios	20
Quinoa	53
Walnuts	15

Dairy and Eggs	Glycemic Index
Butter	0
Cheddar cheese	10
Crème fraîche	50
Eggs	0
Feta cheese	5
Greek yogurt	12
Heavy cream	10
Milk, whole	27
Milk, 1% and 2%	32
Mozzarella cheese	10
Parmesan cheese	5
Plain whole-milk yogurt	20
Ricotta cheese	25
Sour cream	10
Mixed nuts	24

Oil, vinegar, sauces, and condiments	Glycemic Index
Broth, beef, vegetable, and chicken	<10
Coconut milk	10
Coconut oil	0
Cornstarch	87
Cream of tartar	<10
Hoisin sauce	10
Mustard	5
Sambal	10
Soy sauce	10
Tomato paste	40
Vinegar, apple cider	<5
Vinegar, balsamic	10
Vinegar, red wine	0
Vinegar, rice wine	10
Vinegar, sherry	<5
Worcestershire sauce	<5

Sweeteners	Glycemic Index
Brown sugar	68
Carob chips	20
Coconut palm sugar	35
Dark chocolate chips	23
Dark cocoa powder	20
Honey	58

Appendix B

Tips on Grocery Shopping

Shopping Rules

1. Shop around the perimeter of the store. Most grocery stores house fresh, whole food—what we refer to as real food—around the outside perimeter of the store. Typically that's where you'll find the produce, fresh eggs and dairy, and fresh meat, poultry, and seafood. Even the fresh bakery goods are a better option than their packaged counterparts. (While we advocate against sugary desserts, the fresh baked goods are a healthier option should you choose to indulge occasionally.) The center aisles house nearly 20,000 processed packaged, canned, boxed, and frozen items that more often than not should be avoided. These products are often processed into something far different from their original ingredients, and they often have numerous unhealthy ingredients, such as preservatives, added to them.

2. Be label savvy. Read the ingredient and nutrition labels on all food packages carefully. The foods we advise consuming— most often, fresh fruits and vegetables—won't have a label. But anything that does have a label should be scrutinized. Avoid packaged foods that contain more than five ingredients or ingredients that aren't easy to pronounce. Avoid foods that make health claims, such as "low fat" or "sugar free." These are often marketing ploys to entice consumers to purchase products rather than a valid attempt to educate the public about a particular food. For example, a cereal might advertise that it has a third less sugar than before, but that does not give information about the quality of ingredients, or how much sugar still remains.

3. Create a weekly menu, make a shopping list, and stick to your list! Planning a week of meals and making a list of items to purchase specifically for those meals will not only help you create healthier meals, it'll help you budget properly. Do not deviate from your list—if it's not on the list, it doesn't go in your basket!

4. Don't go up and down the center aisles except for items on your list. Leisurely strolls up and down the grocery aisles often cause consumers to fall prey to the previously mentioned marketing ploys. The center aisles do not contain much real, whole food that is essential for our nutrient intake, so go only for the few items that are on your list.

5. Focus the majority of your grocery shopping in the produce aisle. The most nutrient-dense foods are found in the produce department. Using these ingredients as the basis of your meal recipes, as in this book, will ensure you're getting the nutrition that you vitally need. Real foods are healing foods and should be a major staple on your shopping list.

6. Frequent the farmers market. If you're looking for a safe place to leisurely stroll while you shop, head to your local farmers market. Farmers markets are popping up all over the country as more people discover the value of buying fresh, sustainable, local produce. Buying local, seasonal produce directly from farmers is often a less expensive option than shopping at the grocery store, and many farmers use organic growing methods, whether or not they're actually certified as organic.

7. Spend your money wisely. Often people complain that healthy eating and organic produce are too expensive. However, we ask that you complete the following exercise: Sit down with your shopping receipts and take inventory of what you've spent money on. Calculate how much you spent on processed junk food—such as soda, chips, processed meats, and snack items—that have very little nutritional value, and compare the cost to how much you spend on fruits, vegetables, nuts, legumes, and other nutrient-rich foods. If you think healthy eating is expensive, try validating purchases of junk food, which doesn't do anything nutritionally for your body and actually causes harm.

8. Do not go grocery shopping when you are hungry. Going to the grocery store while hungry just invites you to buy things that are not on your list and to choose less healthy options. Going after you've eaten a healthy meal, with a list, ensures that you'll buy just what you need, helping you stick to your health plan and your budget.

9. Follow the 80/20 rule for grocery shopping. Just before you check out, take an inventory of what you're about to purchase. Eighty percent of it should be whole foods and produce, including fruits, vegetables, healthy meats and dairy, nuts, and legumes.

Twenty percent is reserved for packaged foods that are minimally processed. Sticking to this rule ensures that unhealthy stuff isn't wandering into your basket, and that you're able to make healthy meals with the items you've purchased.

10. Have fun! Enjoy your food shopping experience, exploring different foods and learning how healthy choices affect your body. Healthy choices make a healthy you! Ask questions at your local farmers market, and utilize the resources around you. There is so much to learn about food and healthy eating. Make it a fun experience by celebrating the idea of nurturing yourself with healthy, whole foods.

Shopping List

Sometimes people want to make healthy changes and are even ready to do so, but just don't know where to start. Use this shopping list as a guide for building up your pantry and for filling your home with the foods needed to make the healthy recipes in this book.

Don't worry, you don't have to buy everything on the list at once. Start by making a meal plan for the week. Consider what's already in your refrigerator and pantry, then make a list for the additional items that are necessary, particularly the fresh ones. Then add 5 to 10 items to your list to build your pantry. Just add a few if you're stocking up on more expensive items such as certain spices or oils; add more if it's time to get less expensive items like stock, broth, rice, or beans. *Remember always to buy organic when the option is available.*

Greens

- ❑ arugula
- ❑ beet greens
- ❑ chard
- ❑ collard greens
- ❑ endive
- ❑ kale
- ❑ lettuce
- ❑ mustard greens
- ❑ radicchio
- ❑ radish greens
- ❑ spinach
- ❑ turnip greens
- ❑ watercress

Vegetables

- ❑ artichokes
- ❑ asparagus
- ❑ avocados
- ❑ bean sprouts
- ❑ beets
- ❑ bell peppers
- ❑ bok choy
- ❑ broccoli
- ❑ brussels sprouts
- ❑ cabbage
- ❑ carrots
- ❑ cauliflower
- ❑ celery
- ❑ chiles
- ❑ cucumbers
- ❑ eggplant
- ❑ fennel
- ❑ garlic
- ❑ ginger root
- ❑ green beans
- ❑ green onions
- ❑ hearts of palm
- ❑ jalapeños
- ❑ jicama
- ❑ leeks
- ❑ lemongrass
- ❑ mushrooms
- ❑ onions
- ❑ radishes
- ❑ shallots
- ❑ snow peas
- ❑ squash
- ❑ sweet potatoes
- ❑ tomatillos
- ❑ tomatoes
- ❑ turnips
- ❑ zucchini

Fresh Herbs

- ❑ basil
- ❑ chives
- ❑ cilantro
- ❑ dill
- ❑ mint
- ❑ oregano
- ❑ parsley
- ❑ rosemary
- ❑ sage
- ❑ tarragon
- ❑ thyme

Low-Glycemic Fruits
❏ blackberries   ❏ blueberries   ❏ boysenberries

❏ raspberries   ❏ strawberries

Medium-Glycemic Fruits
❏ apples   ❏ apricots   ❏ cherries

❏ coconut (whole or shredded, unsweetened)

❏ grapefruit   ❏ kiwi   ❏ lemons

❏ limes   ❏ melons   ❏ nectarines

❏ passion fruit   ❏ peaches   ❏ pears

❏ persimmons   ❏ plums   ❏ pomegranates

❏ prunes

High-Glycemic Fruits
❏ bananas   ❏ dates   ❏ figs

❏ grapes   ❏ mangoes   ❏ papaya

❏ pineapple   ❏ raisins   ❏ watermelon

Dairy, Meats, and Eggs (Organic, No Added Hormones, Free Range, Grass Fed)
❏ bacon   ❏ beef   ❏ beef, ground

❏ butter   ❏ cheddar   ❏ chicken

❏ cream   ❏ cream cheese   ❏ eggs

❏ feta   ❏ half and half   ❏ milk

❏ mozzarella   ❏ paneer   ❏ Parmesan

❏ Pecorino Romano   ❏ pork   ❏ ricotta

❏ sour cream   ❏ turkey   ❏ turkey, ground

❏ yogurt, Greek

Fish and Seafood

- ❑ abalone
- ❑ albacore tuna
- ❑ black cod
- ❑ catfish
- ❑ char
- ❑ clams
- ❑ cod
- ❑ crabs, Dungeness
- ❑ crabs, stone
- ❑ crawfish
- ❑ halibut
- ❑ lobster
- ❑ mackerel
- ❑ mahi mahi
- ❑ mullet
- ❑ mussels
- ❑ oysters
- ❑ pollock
- ❑ salmon, wild
- ❑ sardines
- ❑ scallops
- ❑ shrimp
- ❑ spot prawn
- ❑ squid
- ❑ striped bass
- ❑ sturgeon
- ❑ tilapia
- ❑ trout, rainbow
- ❑ wreckfish

The fish listed are noted as heart-healthy and low in contaminants.

Grains and Flour

- ❑ barley
- ❑ bread, sprouted
- ❑ bread crumbs (gluten-free)
- ❑ buckwheat
- ❑ cornmeal
- ❑ flour, oat
- ❑ oats, gluten-free
- ❑ oats, rolled
- ❑ pasta, whole wheat
- ❑ rice, brown
- ❑ rice, wild
- ❑ rice, white
- ❑ tortillas, corn
- ❑ tortillas, whole wheat

Beans and Legumes

- ❑ quinoa
- ❑ beans, black
- ❑ beans, cannellini
- ❑ beans, kidney
- ❑ beans, garbanzo (chickpeas)
- ❑ beans, pinto
- ❑ lentils, brown
- ❑ lentils, green
- ❑ lentils, red
- ❑ peanuts, raw and unsalted

Nuts and Seeds (Raw, Unsalted)

- almonds
- brazil nuts
- cashews
- chia seeds
- flax seeds
- pine nuts
- pistachios
- pumpkin seeds
- sesame seeds
- sunflower seeds
- walnuts

Packaged Goods

- adobo sauce
- almond milk, in boxes or cartons
- artichoke hearts
- applesauce, unsweetened
- capers
- chili paste
- clam juice
- coconut milk, in boxes or cartons
- coconut milk, canned
- coconut water
- hoisin sauce
- mustard
- olives
- pumpkin puree
- soy sauce
- tahini
- tomato paste
- tomato sauce
- tomatoes
- white wine

Nut butters (Natural, Raw, Unsalted)

- almond butter
- cashew butter
- peanut butter

Stock and Broth

- beef
- chicken
- vegetable

Oil and Vinegar

- almond oil
- apple cider vinegar
- avocado oil
- balsamic vinegar
- coconut oil
- coconut vinegar
- grapeseed oil
- olive oil
- red wine vinegar
- rice vinegar
- sesame oil
- walnut oil
- white wine vinegar

Herbs and Spices

- [ ] allspice
- [ ] basil
- [ ] bay leaves
- [ ] caraway seeds
- [ ] cardamom pods
- [ ] cardamom powder
- [ ] cayenne
- [ ] chiles, dried
- [ ] chili powder
- [ ] Chinese five-spice
- [ ] cinnamon
- [ ] cloves, ground
- [ ] cloves, whole
- [ ] coffee
- [ ] coriander powder
- [ ] coriander seeds
- [ ] cumin powder
- [ ] cumin seeds
- [ ] curry
- [ ] espresso powder
- [ ] fennel seeds
- [ ] garam masala
- [ ] garlic powder
- [ ] ginger
- [ ] miso
- [ ] mustard seeds
- [ ] mustard powder
- [ ] nori
- [ ] nutmeg
- [ ] oregano
- [ ] paprika
- [ ] pepper, black
- [ ] pepper, white
- [ ] red pepper flakes
- [ ] rosemary
- [ ] saffron
- [ ] sea salt
- [ ] seaweeds
- [ ] thyme
- [ ] turmeric
- [ ] wakame
- [ ] Worcestershire sauce
- [ ] yeast, nutritional

Sweeteners and Baking Products

- [ ] almond extract (unsweetened)
- [ ] almond meal
- [ ] baking powder
- [ ] baking soda
- [ ] carob chips
- [ ] chocolate, dark
- [ ] cocoa powder
- [ ] coconut palm sugar
- [ ] cornstarch
- [ ] cream of tartar
- [ ] honey
- [ ] pure maple syrup
- [ ] molasses
- [ ] peppermint extract (unsweetened)
- [ ] sugar, brown
- [ ] vanilla beans
- [ ] vanilla extract (unsweetened)

Resources

www.glycemicindex.com

nutritiondata.self.com

www.sparkrecipes.com

www.livestrong.com/article/129000-slow-cookers-nutrition

Brand-Miller, Jennie; Foster-Powell, Kaye (2005). *The Low GI Diet Revolution: The Definitive Science-Based Weight Loss Plan.* Marlowe & Company.

Brand-Miller, JC; Stockmann, K; Atkinson, F; Petocz, P; Denyer, G (January 2009). *"Glycemic index, postprandial glycemia, and the shape of the curve in healthy subjects: analysis of a database of more than 1,000 foods."* Am. J. Clin. Nutr. 89(1): 97–105.

Foster-Powell, K; Holt, SH; Brand-Miller, JC (July 2002). *"International table of glycemic index and glycemic load values: 2002."* Am. J. Clin. Nutr. 76(1): 5–56.

Conversions

Useful Conversions

U.S. MEASURE	EQUIVALENT	METRIC
1 teaspoon	--	5 milliliters
1 tablespoon	3 teaspoons	15 milliliters
1 cup	16 tablespoons	240 milliliters
1 pint	2 cups	470 milliliters
1 quart	4 cups	950 milliliters
1 liter	4 cups + 3½ tablespoons	1000 milliliters
1 ounce (dry)	2 tablespoons	28 grams
1 pound	16 ounces	450 grams
2.21 pounds	35.3 ounces	1 kilogram
270°F / 350°F	--	132°C / 177°C

Volume Conversions

U.S. MEASURE	EQUIVALENT	METRIC
1 tablespoon	½ fluid ounce	15 milliliters
¼ cup	2 fluid ounces	60 milliliters
⅓ cup	3 fluid ounces	90 milliliters
½ cup	4 fluid ounces	120 milliliters
⅔ cup	5 fluid ounces	150 milliliters
¾ cup	6 fluid ounces	180 milliliters
1 cup	8 fluid ounces	240 milliliters
2 cups	16 fluid ounces	480 milliliters

Weight Conversions

U.S. MEASURE	METRIC
1 ounce	30 grams
⅓ pound	150 grams
½ pound	225 grams
1 pound	450 grams

Index

About the Authors

Dr. Mariza Snyder is an impassioned and dedicated doctor of chiropractic and wellness practitioner. She currently lives in Oakland, California, where she focuses on helping people to realize their own nutrition and health goals. Dr. Snyder graduated from Life Chiropractic College West in Hayward, California, and began practicing in 2008. She is the coauthor of *The Antioxidant Counter* and *The DASH Diet Cookbook*. In her free time she enjoys staying active, drinking green smoothies and inspiring people to live their best life possible.

Dr. Lauren Clum is a chiropractor committed to helping people achieve their health goals and recognize their own healing capacities. She is the founder and director of The Specific Chiropractic Center in Oakland, California, coauthor of both *The DASH Diet Cookbook* and *The Antioxidant Counter*. After graduating with honors from Life Chiropractic College West, she practiced chiropractic for a year in San Jose, Costa Rica, before returning to the San Francisco Bay Area to open her current chiropractic practice.

Anna V. Zulaica is the founder and chef of Presto! Catering and Food Services. She is the coauthor of *The DASH Diet Cookbook* and her recipes were published in *The Antioxidant Counter*. Anna enjoys cooking and hosting for private parties in the Bay Area, as well as teaching healthy cooking classes and clinics multiple times a year. Her mission is to teach people that healthy cooking can be delicious and that eating healthy is not being on a diet, it is a lifestyle we should all follow.